This is a book about Freedom.

All of us sense that deep inside lies huge potential. We long to experience it, yet something holds us back. We long to set ourselves free, but we don't know how. In this book, you finally learn *how*.

When Brandon Bays was diagnosed with a basketball-sized tumor in her uterus, she was catapulted into an extraordinary, soul-searching journey. Determined to heal naturally, she took no drugs, underwent no surgery; but six-and-a-half weeks later she was declared tumor-free. Going beyond current mind-body wisdom, she discovered a powerful means to get direct access to the soul—the unconditional love, the boundless peace, the living presence within us—and pioneered a revolutionary paradigm for healing. Tens of thousands worldwide have since used THE JOURNEY™ to awaken to their own infinite potential and free themselves from lifelong emotional blocks and physical illnesses.

With practical, easy-to-use techniques, The Journey will enable you to:

- Dive into your own soul and tap into your own inner genius
- Uncover and completely resolve emotional and physical blocks
- Uncover repressed emotions and cell memories that can lead to illness, and clear them
- Heal your being, your emotions, and your body
- Experience the boundless joy, peace, and love within
- Live life as an expression of your highest potential
- Become truly and ultimately free

"An amazing Journey, a gift to us all."
—Jane Seymour, O.B.E., actress, artist, and writer

"Brandon's book is inspiring, exciting and a look deep into the heart about how to live abundantly in a world that often gives too little and takes too much, including the health that sustains us. Her work is a gift to us all."
—Timothy J. Forbess, president, The National Foundation for Alternative Medicine, Washington, D.C.

"Brandon's Journey is a celebration of the new awareness of healing and personal development that is sweeping the planet. It is an inspiration for anyone wishing to liberate themselves and to help them on their path."
—Chris James, award-winning composer, founder of the School for Healing Sound

"The Journey Process developed by Brandon Bays is a deceptively simple technique that facilitates emotional and physical self-healing in the shortest possible time. It can be learned and applied by anyone almost immediately, yet is able to catalyze profound healing results even after other modalities have been tried and failed. I would recommend The Journey Process wholeheartedly to anyone."
—Ian Watson, co-founder of The Lakeland College for Homeopathy, Cumbria, England, and author of *A Guide to the Methodologies of Homeopathy*

"*The Journey* offers a remarkable and innovative approach to accessing important inner resources that can powerfully support the healing of body and mind."
—Walter Jaros, M.D., M.P.H., Chief Medical Officer, Natural HealthLink, and Director of Professional Training, Green Medicine Company

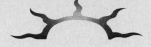

The Journey™

A Practical Guide to Healing Your Life and Setting Yourself Free

Brandon Bays

A Fireside Book
Published by Simon & Schuster
New York   London   Toronto   Sydney   Singapore

In gratitude to
my mother

FIRESIDE
Rockefeller Center
1230 Avenue of the Americas
New York, NY 10020

Originally published in Great Britain in 1999 by Thorsons,
an imprint of HarperCollins*Publishers*

FIRESIDE and colophon are registered trademarks of Simon & Schuster, Inc.

For information about special discounts for bulk purchases,
please contact Simon & Schuster Special Sales:
1-800-456-6798 or business@simonandschuster.com

Manufactured in the United States of America
10   9   8   7   6   5   4

The Library of Congress has cataloged the Pocket Books edition as follows:

Bays, Brandon.
    The journey: a road map to the soul / Brandon Bays.
        p. cm.
    Originally published: Great Britain: Thorsons, 1999.
    1. Spiritual healing. 2. Bays, Brandon. I. Title.

BL65.M4 B39 2001
615.8'52—dc21   2001041428

    ISBN 0-7434-4392-6
        0-7434-4393-4 (Pbk)

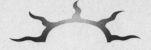

Introduction

This is a book about freedom—freedom to live your life as you've always dreamed it could be.

Deep inside all of us a huge potential beckons, waiting to open us to the joy, genius, freedom, and love within. This presence is calling you home *right now,* longing to set you free. Yet all of us have issues we have felt trapped or limited by. We hear the whispering of our own soul calling to us, but feel unable to access that greatness. Instead, we feel covered or blocked in some way, limited by our issues—anger, fear, depression, grief, hurt, anxiety. It may be as simple as feeling there *must* be something more to life, or as complex as feeling a complete failure. It may be as debilitating as an addiction or as life-threatening as a serious illness.

No matter how deep the issue is and no matter how much you have struggled with it, *the possibility exists for you to become absolutely free, whole, and healed.* You are capable of getting to the *root cause* of these issues, resolving them, letting them go completely, and setting yourself free to live your life at your highest potential, as a full expression of your *true* self.

Through the humbling and profoundly transformative experience of naturally healing from a tumor in only six-and-a-half weeks, I uncovered a boundless joy and freedom that have been my daily experience ever since. This is the most priceless gift of my life. Since that remarkable journey ten years ago, it's been extraordinarily moving and inspiring to watch Journeywork catch fire in every country in which it is offered. Across the globe, tens of thousands of people from all walks of life use Journeywork to discover true freedom in their lives. They're discovering their own answers and uncovering their own deepest truth. They are cleaning out past emotional blocks and physical challenges that have held them back. And they are finally healing on all levels of their being. *Ordinary people are getting extraordinary results.* It seems that no matter what your background is, how old you are, what your culture or upbringing has been, *everyone* knows there is a huge untapped presence inside, and we all secretly long to experience it. This presence is awake while you're asleep at night, making your heart beat, cells replicate, and hair grow. Part of the extraordinary gift of my own healing journey was to discover and pioneer a simple, yet powerful, step-by-step means to get direct access to this infinite wisdom—a wisdom that can reveal to you old emotional patterns and memories stored in your cells, and a healing energy that is capable of resolving and clearing those old issues completely so the body and the being can go about the process of healing naturally.

Today I travel all over the world with Journeywork, giving workshops and advanced programs. I'm always delighted that it attracts people from all the helping professions, both traditional and alternative. I give talks and seminars at hospitals, hospices, abuse centers, homeopathic colleges, healing centers, spiritual organizations, and to cancer support and addiction rehabilitation groups. Everywhere I go, people successfully incorporate Journeywork into their professional programs with ease and grace. I believe we all recognize that there are some issues that simply require more in-depth, roll-up-your-sleeves healing work. We know it's important to address an issue at the *deepest* level to finally clear it out and resolve it completely. Together we understand that Journeywork is a way of bringing about profound healing, wholeness, and a deep sense of well-being—no matter what our backgrounds are. One of the programs I give is a worldwide therapists' accreditation, which has attracted medical doctors, alternative therapists, counselors of all types, psychiatrists, priests, nuns, ministers, social workers—people from all walks of life.

In South Africa, there are doctors taking this healing and forgiveness-based work into communities where they can't afford medical treatments, and we are helping train their staff. Police trauma units are using this work with victims of violent crime. I've trained abuse counselors in Soweto to use the work in their community. In the United Kingdom, Europe, and Australia priests are taking the work back to their flock. A schoolteacher is getting extraordinary results with her youngsters, helping develop the most balanced, confident, high-achieving class in the school. In Australia, where this book is a number-one bestseller, medical doctors and complementary healing therapists keep the book in their waiting rooms for their patients' reference, recognizing that some illnesses require more than just a pill.

Addiction rehabilitation groups are using the work to clear out the intense self-loathing connected with drug abuse, and nurses in cancer treatment facilities are using it alongside the chemotherapy treatments. A swami has taken the work back to his ashram to help people deepen in their experience of the Infinite, and nuns are using it to experience the deep peace within. A rabbi is helping the people in his temple free themselves from long-standing emotional issues, and some therapists who help people on their deathbeds are using Journeywork to open their patients into the infinite peace inside to ease their passing. Journeywork is clearly cross-cultural and appeals to people from all religions, creeds, and walks of life.

What moves me most are the hundreds of phone calls, letters, and e-mails we get from people who haven't had a chance to take the workshops—people who are courageously using the processes explained in this book to undergo their own healing journeys. We hear from people who have successfully and completely cleared long-standing debilitating emotional issues like chronic depression, overwhelming grief, intense low self-esteem, jealousy, abuse, and betrayal. We are always inspired when people share how they've become free from physical challenges including heart disease, breast cancer, chronic fatigue, debilitating arthritis, Crohn's disease, skin diseases—the list goes on. Every day in our office we receive messages of healing from all over the globe. And the message is always the same—*"I was able to tap into my own infinite intelligence, uncover my own blocks, free them, and set myself free—just by using the processes in this book."*

It has been the greatest gift of my life that Grace revealed the means to let go of the past and discover the beauty, love, and peace that is inside all of us. And it's my deepest prayer that *everyone,* not just some of us, awakens to this extraordinary presence of greatness inside, and begins living their life as a full expression of that love, that potential.

This book is written as an expression of the deep gratitude that I feel for the powerful healing process I underwent, with the prayer that it will be a *living tool* that will inspire you to embark on your own journey.

May you discover the boundless joy at the core of your being.

This is your invitation to freedom, your road map to the soul. Are you ready to soar?

"Come to the edge," he said.
"We can't, Master, we're scared."
"Come to the edge," he said.
"We can't, Master, we're scared."
"Come to the edge," he said.
They came.
He pushed them . . .
They flew.

Freedom is our destiny.
Yet we fear taking the very step which will carry us
into the greatness which is our own true nature.

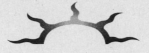

Foreword

I once heard a story that each of us comes into this life as a pristine, pure, flawless diamond. And, through the trials of growing up and the course of life's pains, our innate brilliance becomes hidden by a load of rubbish.

Then, when we become adults, we cover the whole mess with a coat of bright, shiny nail varnish. We present this artificial veneer to the world and wonder why no one seems to think it's that extraordinary. Over time, we may even come to believe that this protective shell is who we really are, and we shape our whole personal identity around it.

But, if we are very lucky, life presents us with a gift—a "wake-up call." Something takes place, when for a moment we crack through the hardened surface, look past the layers of muck, and catch a glimpse of the radiant brilliance shining from deep within.

Then, if we are very, very lucky, we spend the rest of our lives journeying homeward into this exquisite beauty and freedom. We discover that we have *always* been, and will always be, this pristine, flawless diamond.

This is the story of the journey home, and the soul's incessant call for us to recognize the greatness inside ourselves. **It is *your* wake-up call, your invitation to finally come home to whom you really are.**

You are that which you are seeking.

I

I woke up that morning in the summer of 1992 and realized I finally had to face whatever it was that had made my tummy grow so large over the last few months. I just couldn't stay in denial any longer. Some part of me knew there was something seriously wrong inside, and that I was finally going to have to face the doctors and get it checked out.

I didn't want to believe that anything could possibly be "wrong" with me. It seemed I had been doing everything right! I'd been extremely health conscious, proactively conscientious for over twelve years. I ate vibrant, nourishing, vegetarian food, drank only pure, clean, filtered water and rebounded on a mini-trampoline every day. I lived in a little cottage on the beach in Malibu, California, and breathed fresh sea air. More important, because of all the personal growth work I'd done over the years, I no longer needed to direct my thoughts along positive lines; that was already happening naturally. I was deeply fulfilled in my marriage, loved my kids, and felt enlivened by and extremely grateful for my work—traveling the world giving seminars, inspiring others to create vibrant health. My life was everything I had ever longed for.

I'd spent a lifetime attending workshops and seminars, learning everything I could about healing the body and the spirit. It seemed my entire life was about living the principles of health and well-being—I definitely "walked my talk." Yet here I was faced with a tummy so large that I looked pregnant, though I knew I wasn't. How could this be when I was doing everything right?

Embarrassed and ashamed, I couldn't admit my fears to even my closest friends. Here I was, "an expert," teaching others how to take charge of their health, yet I couldn't even zip up my loosest-fitting slacks.

For over fifteen years I had been in the natural healing and alternative health field, and now, faced with a serious health issue, I felt lost at the prospect of going to a "regular" medical doctor. Though I knew I urgently needed a proper medical diagnosis, I had no idea of where to start or whom to call.

Not having the guts to call a friend, and with nowhere else to turn, I decided to check out the local book shop. I scanned the shelves and found a book written by a surgeon who specialized in women's health issues; one who was known for *not* taking out all your organs as the first option. I figured she might be an intelligent place to start, and when I called the number at the back of the book I was surprised and thrilled to get an appointment in only six weeks' time.

During that time, however, it seemed as if my tummy just "blew up" in size, and, oddly, my period began long before it was due. The night before my appointment, I worked up the courage to tell one of my best girlfriends, Catherine, what was going on, and asked her if she would accompany me on my visit.

When we arrived at the doctor's office, I felt sick at the thought of what might be diagnosed. As Catherine and I sat chatting away, waiting to go in for my examination, I broke out in a cold sweat as fear washed through me in waves. After an hour and a half, the nurse finally came and called us in. The forty-five-minute examination was painstakingly thorough and seemed to drag on endlessly. The doctor said virtually nothing as I waited to finally hear what I feared most.

When she finished she quietly turned to me and looked me

straight in the eyes. In a kind but unemotional voice she said, "Brandon, you are equivalent to five months pregnant with a tumor the size of a basketball."

It seemed as if everything started reeling inwardly as I tried desperately to somehow grasp what she had said. I made an awkward attempt at being lighthearted, saying, "Oh come on, Doc, aren't we exaggerating a bit here—a basketball—isn't that a bit over the top? A basketball is this big!" (indicating with my hands the size of a basketball), smiling incredulously and immediately feeling foolish.

Not warming to my attempted humor, she became firm and almost cutting, answering, "Would you rather I called it a beach ball? It's *this* big (indicating a beach ball). And not only that, it's crushing the rest of your organs. Haven't you noticed you've been out of breath lately?"

I nodded and mumbled feebly that I figured it was due to the bloating and weight gain. She said, "It's because this tumor, this 'pelvic mass,' has grown from your pubic area all the way up to your ribcage (touching my body—showing me exactly how much space it occupied) and is pressing against your diaphragm, making it difficult for you to breathe. It's grown so large you need to go into the hospital *today* to have further tests done so it can be surgically removed."

I felt as if someone had knocked the air out of me. I stupidly made a few more feeble attempts at lightening things up before I found the nerve to ask if I could speak to her in her private office.

As we walked down the hall, Catherine was chattering away, firing questions at the doctor. I presumed she was trying to buy me time to pull myself together and get my wits about me. We sat down together, and I asked the doctor what exactly it all meant and what my options were. It seemed the more she talked, the more dire she made things sound. Surgery was my "only option"—and immediate surgery at that.

My heart started to pound as the pressure began to build inside. I felt like a trapped animal. I finally had to come out with it: "I can't let you do that, Doc—I'm in the mind-body healing field. I've got to be given the chance to walk my talk, to try to heal it my own way . . . How much time can you give me?"

She became even more intense and replied that this was not something to take lightly. "You don't understand, Brandon," she said. "It's not just the size of your tumor. My immediate concern is that I could lose you within a few days because of the amount of blood loss you're experiencing. This is not your period. You are bleeding internally."

I began scrambling, negotiating from any angle I could think of. Everything the doctor was saying I was considering intelligently and logically, and I didn't want to do anything to risk my life, but I felt a strong pull—somehow I just *had* to buy myself some more time. I had to have the chance to undergo my own healing process, to give it my best shot.

I asked, "What if I could stop the bleeding through medical hypnosis or homeopathics or something? Then how much time could you give me?" She shook her head in what appeared to be pure exasperation, and dropped into a kind but resolutely firm tone that seemed softly patronizing. She said, "Brandon, you seem like a very sincere person, and I even believe in alternative natural medicine when the diagnosis calls for it, but your pelvic mass is just too big to even consider it."

Indicating the shelves and shelves of books lining her walls as if they were conclusive evidence, she continued, "There is *not one* case history in all these books of a woman who has healed naturally from a pelvic mass the size of yours. So even though you may have the best intent in the world, I can't in good conscience let you out of here in the condition you're in. As a doctor I'm in the business of saving lives, and you need to check into the hospital this afternoon."

"What if you *had* to give me time; how much time could you give me?" I pleaded. And so the negotiation continued, until finally, after another thirty minutes, we reached an agreement that if I could somehow get the bleeding to stop over the next couple of days, I would have one month to do what I knew how to do—to give it my best shot. *If* the symptoms worsened, I would call her immediately, and *if* after one month the pelvic mass was not completely gone, I would come back and let the surgeons do what they knew how to do—remove it surgically.

As I left her office, I looked back into her concerned eyes, and at that moment I saw that she really cared. Yet I could also see that there was no doubt in her mind that I would fail at healing myself. Quietly, with a knowing tone in her voice, she said, "I'll see you in one month's time," absolutely certain that surgery was my destiny.

My heart still pounding, I stepped out into the Los Angeles sunshine and felt that I had been let out of prison. Though I'd never been very fond of L.A., that afternoon somehow it seemed the most beautiful place on earth. The trees seemed to scintillate with color, the air was intensely fragrant, and I felt incredibly lucky just to be alive. My senses were so aware—so keen, so sharp. Life felt so very, very precious.

At that moment something radical happened. It seemed as if time stopped altogether. In that moment, all fear subsided into a deep calm, and a quiet but certain "knowing" arose from within—a knowing that I had been given a big wake-up call and that, in fact, this tumor was a gift—that it had something important to teach me, and that somehow I would be guided to heal myself.

It wasn't even a question of *if* I would heal, but *how*.

Though I didn't know what my healing journey would be, somehow I realized that the same part of me that had been responsible for creating the tumor would also be responsible for *un*-creating it. And in this recognition I felt a childlike innocence and trust that somehow I would be guided to discover what it was this pelvic mass had to teach me.

And so my healing journey began.

2

As I stood in the L.A. sunshine for that brief moment when it seemed as if time stood still, I felt that the whole of my life had been lived to bring me to this very point. Snatches of memories of the various spiritual and mind-body healing teachings I'd experienced through years of study flowed through my mind.

I felt a welling up of gratitude for all I'd learned, for all the teachers I'd learned from, and for all the case histories I'd studied of people who had been diagnosed with illnesses more serious than mine, people who had, with great courage, been successful in healing themselves. Not only had I read, studied, and learned of hundreds of these cases, but also over many years I had been privileged to therapeutically help others as they successfully underwent their healing journeys. I realized that their experiences had been a real-life example for me, and their courage had kindled my own. I knew that if there was just *one* person who had been successful in healing at a physical-cellular level, then it meant that every human body was capable of cellular healing. So I knew without doubt it was possible; I just didn't know what *my* healing journey would be.

I turned around, realizing that I had been immersed in my thoughts for some time, and that my dear friend Catherine was still standing next to me. I gave her a look of incredulity, and said, "Well, at least I've got a month's time. Let's go get some juice. I'm feeling a little shaky—I need to pull myself together."

From the Good Earth health food restaurant I called my husband, Don, who was out of town, giving seminars as Head Trainer with Anthony Robbins. I tried not to let my voice sound overly concerned as I relayed the news—"Remember that appointment I had with the surgeon to check out why my stomach was getting so fat?"

"Oh, yeah, how did it go?"

"Well, I've been diagnosed with a tumor the size of a basketball, and I've been given one month to sort it out."

There was a long silence over the phone—Don was speechless.

Then, "Shit, one month?"

Though an articulate, erudite Ph.D., he seemed utterly at a loss for words. Mumbling something unintelligible he handed the phone over to Tony, who was also *my* boss. I hadn't expected that. I felt very exposed and on the spot, but tried to sound chirpy and confident as I gave Tony the news. Stumbling, I said, "Hey, Tone, I don't know if you'd noticed my stomach has grown kind of fat in recent months." (I thought I'd been successful in covering it up in long, flowing, romantic dresses.)

"Yeah, Brandon, as a matter of fact I had noticed . . ."

Embarrassment washed through me, and I suddenly felt at a loss for words. After a long, awkward pause, all my words came rushing at once—"Well . . . I've been diagnosed with a tumor the size of a basketball, and I've been given just one month to sort it out . . ."

Another long pause seemed to hang in the air, as I waited in anticipation for what I feared would be a humiliating response. But, unexpectedly, he replied in a breezy, encouraging tone, "Not a problem, Brandon, you'll get it handled—I'll see you at Mastery" (a seminar taking place in Hawaii in only one month's time).

Tony passed the phone back to Don, and I gave him a condensed version of all the medical details, assuring him I'd get the blood loss problem handled immediately, and I got off the phone.

I stood by the phone box mildly stunned, mused over the conversation with Tony, and thought about his response. "Not a problem, Brandon, you'll get it handled." I realized the absolute confidence he had in me, and also the certainty he felt about how quickly healing can take place in the body—cellularly. I thought, "He's right, it can and does happen that quickly, and I need to make sure I only tell people who have this knowledge and certainty. I can't afford to invite the negativity of well-meaning people who project their own doubts, fears, and ill-judged sympathy onto me. I've only got one month. *It's precious time.*"

At that moment I made a silent promise to myself that I would tell only those people whom I knew beyond a shadow of a doubt would wholeheartedly support me in a positive way—who were certain that I could and would heal.

I ended up telling only eight people.

After lunch, I immediately went to our local homeopathic pharmacy and spoke to the pharmacist about my condition. He suggested a few herbal and homeopathic remedies, including one to help stop the bleeding, and cautioned me to stop all caffeine intake, as there are statistics that indicate that caffeine can increase tumor size dramatically.

I then went home and did a simple neuro-linguistic mind-body healing process on myself to stop the bleeding. A day and a half later I was surprised and relieved to discover that, except for occasional spotting, the bleeding had stopped.

I then called the doctor. Upon hearing the news, she sounded skeptical but somewhat open, making sure she cautioned me before ending the conversation with ". . . if any of your symptoms worsen at all, call me immediately."

It wasn't until after I put down the phone that I realized I'd actually succeeded in safely buying myself an entire month. I relaxed and breathed a sigh of relief. Then it began to dawn on me that *now* my *real* work lay ahead.

3

In one way I felt an almost childlike curiosity and an openness as to what my journey might bring. And yet I was all too aware that I had been given an urgent wake-up call, and that one month was a very short period of time. I could not afford to squander even one precious moment of it. Though I didn't know where to begin, I felt this constant, insistent inner knowing that somehow I would be guided. So, all I could do was TRUST.

I made a simple promise to myself that I would surrender completely into whatever I was guided to do, and TRUST in wherever that would lead me. I would give it my best shot, no matter what the results. I had no doubt that part of my journey would involve uncovering and discovering what it was the tumor had to teach me. I knew I would need to find out what past unresolved emotional memories and patterns were residing in the cells, learn whatever lessons were there, and finally resolve and release them.

I had the belief, after years of work in the mind-body healing field, that everything happens for a reason and a purpose. Once you learn what the disease or physical block has to teach you and you finally let go of the emotional issues stored in the cells, then, and *only* then, can real healing begin on all levels—emotional, spiritual, and physical. Only then does the body go about the process of healing itself naturally. I knew my journey would have to include letting go of whatever emotional issues were stored inside the tumor. I just didn't know as yet what those issues were.

I also knew I needed to support my body physically in a very practical way if it was to start dumping a huge amount of degenerative and toxic cells! So, the first thing I decided to do was to support my body with a vibrant and clean diet, using well-known natural hygiene therapies I had learned over the years.

I already ate extremely healthful foods, but now I decided to eat in an optimal way, to create the highest levels of energy. I boosted my vegetarian diet from 65 to 70 percent fresh and raw fruits and vegetables to 100 percent completely live food, including lots of freshly squeezed juices. I added food enzymes and increased my mineral intake significantly, and took herbs that I knew would help with the cleansing process. Additionally, I decided to keep my lymphatic system flowing with massage, and my colon cleansed with colonic irrigation, so that when the emotional letting-go was complete, my body would be in top condition to do the physical letting-go. But these were just practical physical supports that were easy to do. I knew my *real* work lay in discovering what was emotionally stored inside that tumor.

Don was in Canada, unable to leave the seminars he was giving. So I decided that day that, given the importance of what was taking place, I should be by his side and that we should take some time out to have a short vacation together, slow things down a bit. Then perhaps the inner guidance might reveal the next step. So I booked a flight to join him in Quebec.

I instinctively knew that my healing journey lay in becoming still, being open, and TRUSTING, TRUSTING, TRUSTING, allowing the next steps to be revealed to me. I somehow understood intuitively that I, the personality of Brandon, was not in charge, but the infinite intelligence inside would be taking the driver's seat. I knew that the part of me responsible for making my hair grow and my heart beat would be doing the work—and that it would take great courage to surrender and relax into the stillness inside, so that the inner guidance could reveal the next step.

So, a little holiday seemed like the best next step.

4

As I sat on the plane to Quebec, I realized I wouldn't be enjoying all the glorious French food there—I'd be dining on crunchy salads and carrot juices and fresh fruit and colloidal minerals. A part of me grew restless and stubborn at the thought; yet I reminded myself I had only a month, and it was the least I could do to support myself.

As Don and I leisurely strolled the quiet, picturesque streets of Quebec, I felt a heightened awareness—my senses seemed so alive and acute. The trees appeared somehow more vibrant, and the smells from the street cafés so varied and full. The cobblestones were rounded from years of people and carriages and cars, and the clouds seemed to stand out vividly against the crisp blue sky. I felt so blessed just to be able to look and smell and feel— even the biting wind seemed somehow rare. It was almost as if my soul itself was tasting life as it *really* is.

A hush fell over me. Once again time seemed to stop. I found myself resting in a sharp stillness that was somehow both utterly unmoving, and scintillatingly alive. The awareness that I was being "guided" arose strongly from within. Outwardly I must have appeared pensive and quiet, but inwardly I was near tears with gratitude for this knowing revealing itself so powerfully.

I looked back at Don; I didn't know how long I had been standing there, but I noticed he seemed unusually quiet. When I probed deeper, Don admitted that he didn't want to share his feelings with me as he knew it was essential for me to be with people who would support me positively with the *certainty* that I would heal, yet he had to admit that he was scared.

"It just seems so big . . ."

Long pause . . .

Quietly I answered, "It *is* big."

I didn't know what else to say. He'd stated the obvious, but somehow the obvious seemed at once incomprehensible and yet so stupidly apparent.

Another long pause . . .

Then I said, "I sometimes get scared, too. And I have to remind myself to be open and trust at those times. No use fighting it. I wish I could somehow explain to you this quiet certainty that keeps coming up from inside, but somehow no matter how worried my mind and personality seem to get at times, something deeper—from within—seems to know different. And this knowing is what is carrying me through this extraordinary journey. So, let's just enjoy our time here, it's such a romantic city." We slipped into a café, and I encouraged him to enjoy the lovely French cuisine, even though I was only eating salad. Reluctantly, he agreed.

Day by day the peace deepened, and after three or four days in Quebec I knew it was time to move on. To what, I still didn't know, but something inside seemed to be urging me onward.

5

From Quebec I decided to give our friends Mark and Elaine Thomas a ring. They were living in a spiritually based community in upstate New York, and I figured I could visit them, have some good bodywork done, and get their advice on what to do next. It was with Mark and Elaine that Don and I had undergone much of our training in natural hygiene, iridology, acupressure, herbal healing, and so on, as well as a process called body electronics. Mark and Elaine had seen us both through a time of great spiritual and emotional transformation in our lives, and even though it was years later and we'd moved on to different aspects of mind-body healing, somehow they seemed to be the right people to be around. I knew they'd be supportive.

When we arrived, Elaine offered us all a cup of herbal tea, and said in her forthright and intuitive style, "So what's up? Something's going on!"

"Well, I've been diagnosed with . . ."—I laid the whole story out, including the physical things I was doing, and finished by saying, "So I'm letting myself be guided."

Shrugging, she said, "Brandon, I don't even see this as an issue. You're going to get this handled . . . no problem . . . it'll be a breeze. . . . I just know it. . . . Really, I mean it, Brandon." And I knew she did.

Once again someone was hearing the news for the first time and using the *exact words* Tony did—"No problem, you'll get it handled." It was beginning to feel like the people around me were a mirror of that same inner knowing that was arising in me! The outer confirmation of what I felt inwardly to be true was somehow very reassuring.

I did manage to get some good massage bodywork while I was there, and also found a herbalist who suggested several herbs to aid in the cleansing process. As I prepared to leave, the massage therapist handed me a small slip of paper with a phone number. "I did some research for you and found a good cranial-visceral massage therapist in Santa Monica. That's not far from Malibu, is it?"

"No, just down the road," I replied. "Thanks, that was very kind of you."

"Not to worry, Brandon—I really see this thing leaving you easily. You'll get it handled."

There it was again—third time! This time my hair stood on end. It really was beginning to feel as if the universe was trying to tell me something. If I ever believed in such a thing as a sign, then I was getting signs from all over the place, and they were all pointing to the *same* thing—YOU'LL GET IT HANDLED!

Holding the slip of paper, I thought, "Hmm, maybe this guy is one of the bread crumbs, the signposts along my path. I'll give him a ring as soon as I get back to Malibu."

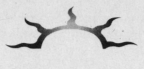

6

On my way home from the airport, holding the slip of paper in my hand, I felt an unexpected anticipation building. I could barely wait to see where this new signpost would take me next.

With a spring in my step I bounded through my front door in Malibu, reached for the phone, dialed the number on the slip of paper, and got the massage therapist's secretary. She apologized profusely, but he didn't have a single opening for one month. Did I want to schedule for then?

A month? I didn't have a month! I had less than three weeks left.

I felt as if someone had stuck a pin in my balloon. How could it be that he couldn't see me? I was just so *sure* he was part of my journey—one of my signposts. So far everything had flowed so perfectly, so gracefully—as if I was somehow in "the zone" that so many athletes speak of. This couldn't be right. I asked her if she was absolutely certain.

"Yes, I'm sorry—he's completely booked."

Deflated, I put the phone down, still somehow unconvinced. Two minutes later I redialed—"Could I at least speak to him?"

"He's with a client."

"Well, could you pass on my message?"

"I'll let him know you called."

That night at 10:45 I received a phone call beginning with a flurry of apologies for calling so late. "My name is Benjamin—I'm the cranial-visceral massage therapist you phoned."

We talked until 11:00 P.M., and he said, "Listen, if you don't mind coming at 7:00 A.M. I'll fit you in for as many sessions as I can between now and your time to go back for tests. Can you make it that early?"

"I can't afford not to. I'll be there at 6:45."

Though early mornings have never been my best times, I was thrilled to be actively working toward physically healing myself, and glad that things once more seemed back "in the flow" and on track.

At the end of the first session, Benjamin turned to me as I reached for my coat, and said, "You know, I don't get the feeling that this is really going to be a problem for you; I almost get the feeling it's already healing itself. I know it sounds crazy, because your examination is less than three weeks away, but I get the feeling you are going to get this thing handled!"

I practically repeated it out loud with him! What was this, a mantra? I shook my head, smiled, and waved goodbye—"See you tomorrow."

Benjamin had given me the name of a very good colon therapist. I promptly followed this up, and got an immediate appointment. During our colonic session she felt around my belly and said, "You know, I get the feeling this is going to move out very quickly, but there's some old emotional stuff stored in there that you need to let go of."

"I know," I mumbled quietly. I was already all too aware that although I was actively taking care of my physical body in preparation for the healing, I still had not yet addressed the emotional side—I had not got to the core of what created the tumor in the first place. I checked inside to see if I was avoiding facing the issue, and I honestly didn't feel I was. I was just staying open and trusting I would be guided, and I hadn't yet felt "called" or pulled to dive into the emotional cause of the tumor.

It took a lot of courage, and more patience than I was normally accustomed to, to keep trusting, as I was fully aware that time was marching on! That night I got a phone call from my dear spiritual friend, Kabir, in San Francisco. He is an oncologist, a doctor who specializes in cancer, and I listened as he gave an hour's earful of technical medical detail, most of which I didn't fully understand. I kept feeling, "There's got to be a reason I'm listening to all this." Finally, toward the end of the conversation, he got out of doctor mode and back into friendship mode, and I was able to get a word in edgewise. I let him know that it was not my intention to go the orthodox medical route. I intended to try healing on my own before giving the surgeons a chance to cut me open, and I really wanted to get at the emotional issues that I knew were at the core of it all, and get the learning that this pelvic mass had to give me.

"Brandon, I just got an idea! You should come visit me for a couple of days; I've got this great bodyworker who helps people let go of the emotional issues stored inside while working on your body—it's fabulous work. I go there myself about once a week. She's magic! I really have got a lot out of her sessions."

For a doctor, sometimes he sounded so dramatic, but something in what he said called to me, and besides, even if she wasn't that brilliant, I could always go over to the local meditation center there, meditate, and attend some programs—plus I'd get a chance to hang out with Kabir and have some of our spiritual chats.

"I'll see if I can get good flights. If not, then we'll assume it's not meant to be."

As grace would have it, I got one of those super-duper special discount deals on two tickets to San Francisco only forty-eight hours later. It was only two and a half weeks before I had to reappear at the doctor's office and here I was once again— TRUSTING, TRUSTING, TRUSTING!

I was delighted to find Kabir had already organized a couple of appointments for me. Being a doctor, he himself had next to no time to see me, which suited me fine as I had a feeling when I stepped off the plane that something important was going to happen in San Francisco.

I made an uncharacteristic decision *not* to go to Kabir's home, but to book Don and me into a great little bed-and-breakfast inn just down the street from the therapist. Figuring I had only a few short days there, I thought I might like to rest between sessions and keep quiet and let myself heal. Plus, the bed-and-breakfast was virtually down the street from the meditation center, where I could go to meditate and sit in silence.

Some part of me instinctively knew that the time had come to face the music—to turn inward and keep to myself. I didn't know how important that decision would turn out to be.

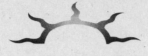

7

As I went up the steps to meet Surja, the massage therapist, something inside began to feel wobbly and a little scared. I wondered what that was all about, and dismissed it as I rang the bell.

A lady with a kind face answered. With very reassuring tones, she took me to her treatment room, which was warm and clean and somehow nurturing in a simple, homey way. I asked her what the teddy bears on the chair were for. "Oh, for kids when they come here. It makes them feel secure. Some adults like them too." I smiled, and got the feeling that they were there mostly for the adults. It seemed a little quaint, but sweet, just the same.

She was burning some fragrant incense, and had pictures of a couple of spiritual masters she had studied with. Though massage was her speciality, I could see she had a great love of Spirit, and probably had the same thirst for learning that I do.

We got to chatting before we started, and I told her the whole story from beginning to end—that it was my firm belief that emotional memories are stored in the cells of the body and get passed on from one cell generation to the next, and that real healing begins when you let go of these cellular memories. I prayed, with all my heart, to finally face whatever was stored inside that tumor. I hoped she could help.

I admitted to her that, being in the mind-body field myself, I'd probably tried and done *everything* over the past twenty years. I felt I'd experienced every healing technique available, and figured I'd already handled all my emotional issues. So, when my belly kept growing and growing, it never occurred to me that there could actually be something seriously wrong. I had to admit that perhaps I'd grown arrogant—thinking it couldn't happen to me.

I let her know something that I hadn't shared with anyone else—how humbling it had been, and how ashamed I'd felt not only to find out how large the tumor had grown, but also to realize how long I'd stayed in denial. I just hadn't wanted to believe that anything could be wrong with me, as I was supposedly doing everything right.

She stopped me to say, "You know, it sounds like you *were* doing everything right—it just seems to me like this must be some *old* stuff you need to get rid of."

"But I feel like I've done every healing process on the planet!"

"Well, clearly your body doesn't think so! The fact that your emotional stuff has manifested at the physical level must mean that *you're finally ready to face it and let it go.*"

I knew she was right, and nodded in quiet agreement. It seemed apparent that we shared the same beliefs about health, and I felt very comfortable.

We continued swapping stories of various therapeutic practices, and laughed at some of the more ridiculous things we'd tried when we were younger. Then we began sharing our different spiritual realizations. About forty-five minutes slipped away before we both realized we were taking up precious therapy time.

Before we started I made a silent prayer that I would have the courage to face whatever was stored inside that tumor. I then opened and surrendered inwardly, and allowed myself to expand into the stillness that had been my constant companion throughout my journey. I knew instinctively it was definitely from the stillness that all the answers would come—*not* from my personality, and certainly *not* from my chattering mind. If my *thinking* mind was to have come up with the answers, it surely would have done so by now. As it hadn't, my only route was trust: trust in a *deeper* wisdom, the wisdom responsible for making my heart beat, my eyes shine, my hair grow; trust in the infinite intelligence responsible for making my cells replicate; trust in the part of me that is awake when I'm asleep at night. I knew I would have to trust and surrender into my very essence—into the real me—into what felt like "home" to me.

As she began massaging me, I closed my eyes and felt myself relaxing ever more deeply into peace, and once again I had the experience of time standing still—my senses fully alive, and yet my mind completely at rest, with a presence of peace that seemed vast, without boundaries. I felt myself connected with everything.

While massaging, Surja suggested, "Why don't you, in your mind's eye, take some steps right down into your tumor and see what it looks like down there?" Her suggestion seemed so obvious, but somehow it felt right. So I decided to do just that.

When I got inside my uterus I didn't like what I saw. It was pretty scary-looking, and more than once I thought, "I'm getting out of here. I don't want to see all this." But my inner wisdom kept reminding me that I was here for a reason, and so once again I prayed for the courage to face whatever it was I needed to face. I was certain I was going to find something I just couldn't bear to see.

As I was "walking about" inside the tumor, I came to an area that seemed particularly dark. As I approached the area, I could sense an intense feeling of fear emanating from the walls. Spontaneously, an old memory of an intense childhood trauma flashed before me. Instantly, my doubting, thinking mind checked in and said, "It can't be that—I know all about that memory— I've long since dealt with that issue and put it to bed! It wasn't *that* big a deal—it can't be the cause of what's going on in here . . . blah . . . blah . . . blah . . ."

As Surja continued to massage, I shyly relayed the judgments my thinking mind was making. She said reassuringly, "Well, your body wisdom is probably coming up with that particular memory for a reason. For now, why don't you just go with what's coming up for you? Even if your *thinking* mind is doubting it, what have you got to lose?"

And so I continued watching the memory. In my mind, I found myself going through the scene as if in living color, and in slow motion. Surprisingly, unexpected emotions that I had buried and long since forgotten seemed to be arising, and the true expression of how I felt at the time seemed to be surfacing. I hadn't realized how intensely I had really felt. I'd been too successful, even then, at masking my true emotions by putting on a brave face.

Tears quietly streamed down my cheeks.

I felt very private, and I didn't want to say much to Surja about it. And yet, there was a great relief in finally just being real with myself—taking the mask off and letting myself experience the incredible vulnerability and helplessness that I felt as a young child in that memory. I was finally letting myself *feel* the natural emotions that I hadn't let myself experience at the time of the trauma. Somehow, even as a small child I'd learned that I wasn't allowed to show my true feelings. And, more important, I hadn't been able to admit them to myself.

So, in a very simple, pure way I was finally allowing myself to experience what had been there all along. I had never really forgotten this old memory, and the "discovery" of it was no real revelation. What came as a surprise was the *intensity* of my *true* feelings—I'd been so successful in putting a lid on them that I managed to convince myself that it wasn't that important!

I shared a little of what I was going through with Surja, and gently she asked me, "Do you feel complete?" I checked inside with the inner wisdom. "No."

"Well, why don't you imagine a little campfire, and put all the people in your memory there with you; and why don't you have a fireside chat and find out why the other people were behaving as they did, and let them know your true feelings—let the younger you talk to them as if they were here right now."

Once again, what she said seemed like a good idea, so I thought

I'd give it a go—I had nothing to lose. Meanwhile, I was still getting a lovely relaxing massage. Surja seemed to instinctively know in which area I was carrying tension, and she would ease it as I carried on with my internal processing.

Inside my mind's eye, I pictured myself at a crackling campfire. Both my parents were there—they looked so much younger, and dressed in the corny style of the 1950s—and the four-year-old me who'd gone through the emotional memory was standing there in her little dress, looking very unprotected and unsure of herself. The present me was also there, so I decided to go over to the younger me and invite her to sit in my lap, so that she could feel safe and comforted.

I was very surprised at what was said at the campfire. I hadn't realized how intensely the younger me had felt about this old memory. It seemed the little me had a lot of unexpressed pain to share.

She finally said what she had been unable to say for years. It seemed as if years of pain poured out of her. When she seemed empty of words, I turned to my parents and asked why they had behaved as they did. I was equally surprised to hear what was going on for them at the time, and tears of compassion sprang to my eyes as I finally understood the source of their pain, and how frustrated and helpless they felt. My sister had drowned at the age of four, and unfortunately their inexpressible pain would sometimes spill out and get directed at the rest of us.

The fireside chat continued until we'd all finally emptied ourselves out, having shared from our deepest hearts. And my little childhood self finally, for the very first time, truly understood why and how everything had taken place. I was left in peace— peace, simplicity, and true understanding.

I related a very condensed version of what had taken place to Surja, and she asked me once again if I finally felt complete with this old issue. I checked inside. "No, there's something still niggling me inside, but I don't know what it is—it's just a feeling that something else still needs to take place."

I felt at a loss. I knew there was no sense in turning to my thinking mind. It would only give me some obvious logical-seeming answer that had already been unsuccessful in helping me to heal, or it would judge me and tell me how stupid this all was.

So, once again I felt myself opening and trusting and surrendering into the silence—I knew the answers would come from there. As the silence became very vast, very pervasive, my thinking mind was arrested and, once again, I felt awed by the beauty of the peace that seemed to be emanating from my soul. My thoughts came to rest, as silence seemed to fill the room.

From the depths of the silence, I heard the words (or rather somehow experienced them)—"You need to forgive your parents."

It hit me like a stone. I knew it was the truth. It was so obvious, but it had never occurred to me before. So, in my mind's eye, I reconstructed the campfire and put my parents by the fire. Then, inwardly, the younger me forgave both of them—in the innocent way that children forgive. I felt as if my heart was breaking as the words of forgiveness came from my lips. The forgiveness was absolutely authentic, and came from the very depths of my soul.

Tears streamed down my cheeks. Peace washed through my body, the peace of completion. A simple knowing arose from within, a knowing that THE STORY WAS OVER!

As I lay there on the massage table, I began to feel a subtle but palpable energy coursing through my arms and legs, then throughout my whole body. Somewhere deep within I knew the tumor's healing had begun.

After a short while, Surja gently let me know that it was time for the session to end. Two hours had gone by. It had seemed so much quicker than that! Gently, I sat up, feeling a little light-headed, and she handed me a glass of water.

She suggested that I might like to go back to the bed-and-breakfast, maybe have some soup, take a rest, and just allow things to continue to process inside. I nodded silently—I didn't feel much like talking—and quietly prepared to get down off the massage table.

Inwardly, my doubting, thinking mind had slowly crept back, and was now in full force saying things like, "This wasn't that big a deal—so you found an old memory—so what? . . . You've done this kind of thing before. . . . Been there, done that, got the T-shirt. . . . All this was just in your mind, in your imagination. . . ." and on, and on.

I slipped off the table, my mind chattering away, and reached for my clothes. As I put my arm out to grab my slacks, I felt wildly off balance, woozy and wobbly all over. I had to grab for a chair to sit down.

In that instant my mind stopped all criticism, and quietly turned all of its focus to what was going on in my body. I thought, "Shit!—something is happening here—something big!" and I reached down to touch my taut-as-a-drum belly to find it had actually gone just a tiny bit soft! I thought, "I must be dreaming—things can't happen this quickly." My mind began to race—it couldn't comprehend what was taking place. I felt sick all over. All I wanted to do was lie down.

Don was already out in the living room, waiting for me, and I didn't want him to see how sick I was feeling. I felt extremely disoriented—I could feel that things inside were shifting rapidly, but if I had to explain what I meant by that, I knew I couldn't.

Gently, I made my way into the car. When I got to my room at the bed-and-breakfast, I was unbelievably grateful to slip into the clean white sheets and just snuggle down and rest, while whatever it was that was taking place, took place.

I continued "processing" through the day, and during the night I slept fitfully. I woke up the next morning feeling weak and vulnerable, uncomprehending. Everything was happening so quickly. It felt as if the molecules in my body were buzzing and shifting, and when I touched what had been my hard, pregnant-feeling tummy, it felt like jelly.

For three days I was weak and disoriented. I felt somehow raw and exposed, as my body seemed to go about the process of doing what it knew how to do. I was absolutely certain of one thing. "I" wasn't in charge—my body wisdom had powerfully taken over and was transforming my cells naturally and perfectly, of its own accord, without me having to think about a thing.

Strangely, my mind finally shut up—it had no more judging comments to make. The fact that things were working perfectly well without its interference was so powerfully evident, it had nothing more to say about it. I rested in a peace that was all enveloping. I felt very childlike, innocent, completely content *not* to understand any part of what was taking place internally. I just rested easily in the sweet, all-embracing acceptance that was present. The intelligence of the body wisdom was working its own miracle inside, and all I could do was rest in gratitude and surrender.

As I rested in quiet contemplation, it occurred to me that all along I had thought this tumor was clinging to me, when in fact *I* had been clinging to *it*—protecting myself from the memory and painful feelings stored there. And when I finally discovered the emotional patterns and memory connected to it, and finished the story, that's when the need for the tumor finally finished. Once the issues were completed, healed and forgiven, the tumor was able to leave. It had fulfilled its purpose and given me its teaching.

It seemed as if I had literally put the painful memory into a package, and put a lid on it. Then the cells had grown and grown to keep the old memory encapsulated, protecting me from having to face it over the years. Or so it seemed, looking back on it.

8

It was now only ten days until I was due back at the doctor's office. Daily, my stomach was growing flatter, although as I got close to the due date I could see it was not yet completely flat.

By this time I was already back in Malibu, and I decided to see if I could accelerate my healing. I asked a few of my closest friends to help me go through the memory processing two more times, although this time, instead of massaging my body, they held acupressure points relating to my internal organs.

Once again, I surrendered deeply into the silence, and spontaneously the inner knowing brought up a few more memories—different ones from the first, but all centered on the same theme. I found I was forgiving myself, as well as the other people involved, but I could see I was just learning different aspects of the same lesson.

It was as if there was one *core issue* and I had spent a lifetime repeating the same pattern, making the same painful mistakes, but with different people. It was as if I had a string of memories that was like a pearl necklace—even though each memory or each pearl had a slightly different shape, size and hue, they were all essentially the same. And it felt to me that on that day with Surja, we had broken the string, and now all the pearls were just sliding off—all the memories were just finishing themselves and leaving. When we were done with each process I felt profound shifts and movement that continued for several hours.

Two days before my doctor's appointment, I kept feeling my tummy. It had gone down in size dramatically, but it still didn't feel completely flat. So, when I sat in the doctor's office, waiting for my examination, my heart began to pound. I felt a mixture of excitement, anticipation, and fear washing through me; my knees felt weak and my hands sticky. Once again I sat there fearing the worst, waiting for the doctor to lower the boom.

Once again, we went through a thorough examination, only this time the doctor talked to me as it was progressing. She mentioned that she had sent the previous test samples in to discover whether the mass was malignant or benign, but they had been contaminated with all the blood, so she was going to have to redo the tests. I kept thinking, "I don't want to hear about the previous tests. Just tell me what's going on *now.*"

As she was speaking, I suddenly remembered that a year earlier I had Pap smear results that had come up as precancerous. On a scale of one to five, with five being cancerous, I was a three. At the time I didn't really give it any thought, as my alternative healthcare practitioner had dismissed the result, saying that many things could contribute to a precancerous smear result—even a vaginal infection. So, I had just let it go. I realized now that I ought to have investigated it further.

Finally, the doctor said, "Well, there's been a big improvement. The pelvic mass seems to have gone down significantly—from the size of a basketball to the size of a six-inch cantaloupe melon."

The words fell on my ears with a dull thud.

"A six-inch cantaloupe—are you sure it's still that big?" I said. Disappointment filled me.

"That's a dramatic change, Brandon—it's gone all the way down from pushing against your diaphragm, three inches above your waistline, to right here, two inches *below* your waistline. I can cup my hand right around the top of it. Here, touch it with your own hand—can you feel it?"

"Yeah," I said, trying to fight back tears.

"Think of a basketball." (She showed me with her hands.)

"Now think of a six-inch cantaloupe melon. (She showed me again.) That's a significant change." Long pause. "But it's not significant enough, Brandon. You still need to have it surgically removed."

I turned my face away so she couldn't see me as I wiped my eyes, and quietly asked if we could talk about it in her consultation room. I thought it had gone down a *lot* more than that. As I sat with her, her words seemed to come through a haze. She clearly could see I was upset and was trying to assuage me while remaining firm in outlining the direction I should take.

"It's a huge improvement, Brandon. There's nothing to be disappointed about. Clearly you've been doing something to heal yourself. But I feel I must let you know tumors are known to be volatile, and it is possible for them to vacillate radically in size— that's why your tummy blew up in size in the six weeks before your first visit. There's nothing to say it won't blow up in size again. You need to get real about this, Brandon. You need to get the tests done to determine its nature, and once they are complete, have it surgically removed. That's my strong advice to you. This is not something to take lightly."

Everything she said made sense from a logical point of view. But everything inside me was still saying NO! I sat there quietly as she spoke, not offering any outward resistance—just trying to take on board her words, and truly weigh their validity. There was no doubt she made sense. But that inner knowing of "you'll get it handled" was still strongly in the background.

At one point, in a mildly disinterested voice, she asked what I had done over the last month for such a dramatic change to take place. I piped up, hoping that she might actually want to hear about the intense emotional healing journey I'd undergone. Innocently, with great enthusiasm I began to launch into my story. She stopped me short.

"No, no! I just want the facts. What have you been *doing physically*? What foods have you been eating? What herbs, if any, have you been taking? Has your diet changed significantly? What about your physical activity? I just want the *facts* for my file."

So I began listing out all the herbs, enzymes, colloidal minerals, colonics and massages, and ended by saying that I was on 100 percent fresh and raw fruits and vegetables, combined with fresh squeezed juices.

She noted it all down, closed the file, and said dryly, "Well, you may have to remain a raw food-ist for the rest of your life, if you think that's what created the change"—with a wry, sardonic smile that looked unbecoming on her otherwise pretty face.

Inwardly, a door slammed. I stopped feeling like a helpless wimp and got it: this was not a doctor who wanted the *whole* picture, the *real* facts, which included the emotional side of things. She wanted *her* idea of what the facts were! I realized there was no further basis for discussion, and something inside said ENOUGH.

Simply, and somewhat curtly, I thanked her for her time, and said that my belief was not that the tumor would blow up and down and up again, but that I was on a healing journey. I was determined to honor my body, and would give it whatever time it needed to complete the healing process.

She looked dumbfounded. She became very unattractive as she attempted to persuade me that I was in dreamland, and reiterated that my only option was surgery. I looked at her as I left, and felt a strange combination of compassion and disgust—is healing only about the food we eat, and the medicine we take? I realized that that was simply her model of the world, and that it wasn't her fault—her training was necessarily narrow. Doctors are trained to work on bodies—in the same way that mechanics are trained to work on cars. They go into the healing field ostensibly to help people heal, but somewhere along the way they forget that people aren't just their bodies. We *have* bodies, minds, and emotions, but most importantly what we *are* is *soul*—something that can't be touched, tested, or surgically removed.

As I drove home, I was very glad for the wake-up call her lack of understanding had given me. Her arguments had been very seductive, and I had begun to fall into a doctor's idea of how to heal someone—you fix them by taking out the parts. It took her total lack of interest in the rest of my healing journey to make me realize once again that I must follow my own truth no matter how foolish it appeared from the outside. It was a hard choice, because unlike attacking the tumor from a purely physical level, you couldn't see, touch, or even "test" the emotional shifts that had taken place inside me; and yet, for me, they were every bit as real as the physical shifts that seemed to follow from them as a direct result.

At that moment I felt very alone. Logically, I knew it wasn't true, as I had devoted, supportive friends and family, yet somehow I still felt lonely. I realized that there is a way in which everyone must follow their own, unique healing path, and it is an experience that no one else can have for you. Spiritual transformation is an inner journey—it's the soul's personal path of learning and letting go, and it's something that must be experienced on your own.

9

When I stepped through the door, there was a message on the answering machine from Don, who was in Hawaii preparing for a Tony Robbins two-week seminar called Mastery. He had remembered my appointment with the doctor and was wondering how it had all gone—he sounded enthusiastic and supportive. I really felt I needed to talk to him, to share what was going on, but felt inwardly ashamed—that somehow I'd failed—it hadn't completely healed.

At the thought of Don and my friends in Hawaii, I felt even more alone. Some of my closest friends were there. I didn't want anyone to know—I knew they were rooting for me and would be very disappointed. I knew I needed to give it more time.

Then I remembered my first conversation with Tony—"No problem—you'll get it handled, I'll see you at Mastery." I hadn't made it to Mastery. My failure was so clearly obvious.

Tony's wife, Becky, had sweetly called me three days earlier, warmly imploring me to come along to Mastery—"You don't have to work—you could just come and hang out—be there in support of Don." I'd been touched by her reaching out to me, but quietly answered, "Beck, it means so much to me that you would call, but this is one time I need to give myself completely into my own healing journey. I've been there for so many people over the past thirteen years. Right now is just not the time for me to give to others, even if I'm just in the background. I've promised myself that for once I'd just support me, and I'd give it my best shot." These were hard words for me to say, as my whole heart and soul wanted to be there to help, yet I knew I had to keep my promise to myself.

I knew Don wouldn't be available to talk to until late that night, so I decided to give my dear friend Skip a call, to confess my "failure" to somebody and at least get it off my chest. He'd been one of the eight people I'd shared my healing journey with, and had been there with me from the beginning. He'd held my acupressure points for both sessions as I'd continued my processing, and had really seen me through an intense and powerful transformation. He'd been irrepressibly supportive all along, and I figured he might help me lighten up, at the very least.

Skip answered the phone with his normal enthusiasm. "Hey, Brandon! How'd it go?"

"Well, not as well as I'd hoped. It only went from the size of a basketball to the size of a six-inch cantaloupe." I related the whole doctor's visit.

"Hey! Hey! Stop right there, Brandon. Did you say it went from a basketball to a cantaloupe? That's incredible . . . you're amazing! What are you worried about? It's on its way down. Don't listen to what that doctor told you—just look at the *results*. You *know* it's *not* going to blow up and blow down—YOU KNOW what created that shift—I was there with you when most of it happened."

Then, chastisingly, as if speaking with humor to a child, he said, "You know better than this. This isn't the Brandon I know! LOOK WHAT YOU'VE DONE. IT'S ON ITS WAY OUT, BRANDON!!! It's just a matter of time—give it a week or two. At the rate it's moving, your stomach will be flat in *no time!* What are you thinking?"

His unbridled enthusiasm, coupled with his absolute certainty that I would heal, and his incredulity at my state were contagious, and made me laugh at myself. Sheepishly, I had to admit he was probably right.

"Well, Skipper, it's just hard to stay strong when a doctor's in your face basically telling you you're full of shit."

"*She's* full of shit!" he said with a warm, "I don't mean it" kind of laugh. "She doesn't know the intensity of what you've gone through, or the surrender and trust it's taken for you to really look at those old outmoded dinosaur issues that were lurking inside that tumor. She doesn't know how free you've become. You're radiant, Brandon. Look at yourself in the mirror. Give me a break!"

His enthusiasm won me over, hands down.

"Dump that doctor, Brandon. She doesn't know who you are. She doesn't know what you are capable of. Listen, my wife is going to an incredible doctor here at Cedars Sinai hospital. Why don't you give them a call and see if you can get an appointment, say in two weeks? Your tumor's gotta be gone by then. You know Cedars—it's one of the best in the country. They've got this incredible high-tech equipment they've been using with Jill (his wife, who was having complications with her pregnancy), and they are really caring. Want me to give them a ring? They are *state-of-the-art*, Brandon. You should get it checked out by the best. You should put your mind at rest."

Hesitatingly, I said yes—wondering if the tumor would actually be gone by then.

"I'll call you right back. I'll see what I can do."

Five minutes later he called back, all excited—"Hey, I got you an appointment not this Wednesday, but next. You're gonna love their office, everyone's really nice. You might have to wait a couple of hours because they seem to get really booked, but I promise you it'll be worth it."

Over the next week and a half I was delighted to see Skip's words about the tumor going down in size coming true. My stomach grew flatter and flatter as the week went on. When I went to my massage therapist, he kept insisting, "Brandon—I just get the feeling there's nothing there. I can't feel it with my hands anymore, no matter how deeply I dig in."

My colon therapist echoed his sentiments, saying that she intu-itively sensed I'd let go of years of emotional baggage. And throughout the time, I continued taking the herbs, eating only fresh and raw fruits and vegetables, drinking loads of freshly squeezed juices, taking the minerals, and supporting my thinner and more vibrant-growing body the best I knew how.

10

The following Wednesday, when I showed up for my appointment, I felt quietly excited, a little scared, and innocently hopeful. Skip was right—I had to wait over two hours as the waiting room seemed in constant flux with expectant mothers and mothers with babies. I tried to interest my racing mind with the various magazines around, but found I was too restless with anticipation.

Finally, a nurse came and called my name, and I was ushered past several open doors through which I could see all kinds of complex-looking equipment. The nurse asked me to change, as she proudly explained the various pieces of equipment in the room I was waiting in. "It's the latest technology—with it the doctor can quite accurately see inside your organs. If you want she'll turn the monitor screen toward you so you can watch what she is doing. You'll find the doctor very helpful—she'll explain everything to you as she takes the pictures. If you want, we've got the latest thing—pregnant mothers just love it—it's a machine which can develop the pictures within moments of the times they are taken. It's like a Polaroid—pregnant mothers like to take them home to show off the baby *in utero*. If you want, just ask the doctor—she'll give you yours."

I thought how technical it all seemed, but I warmed to the nurse's obvious friendliness, and when she left my heart began to pound as I sat there in the cold equipment-filled room, waiting for the doctor to arrive.

Five minutes later she breezily walked through the door, not wearing the standard doctor's coat. Immediately I liked her. We chatted together about what a nice couple Skip and his wife Jill were, and finally got around to the purpose of my visit.

I had already made the decision that I would not tell my whole story to this doctor. I wanted a fresh *unbiased* opinion based on technical results, not on the diagnosis of my previous doctor. So I got around it by saying, "I'm thirty-nine years old, and my gynecologist thought it would be a good idea to get a complete ultrasound examination—she was concerned I might have a small growth, and as I'm the age for such things to occur . . ."

She interrupted me to ask, "In the uterus, the ovaries—where?"

"She didn't actually say," trying to remain vague and noncommittal.

"Well, why don't we do a comprehensive exam? We'll get the whole picture that way. There is a new piece of equipment that we recently acquired that makes it so much more accurate and easy to see. It may not be as comfortable, because it means I'm going to have to put a probe up inside you, but I promise I'll be gentle. This way we'll go at it from all angles."

I answered I was actually quite eager to be as clear and thorough as possible, and would willingly cooperate with whatever she thought was necessary. The examination went much as the nurse had said it would. The doctor was very chatty, and clearly did her utmost to put me at ease while dealing with a very clinical, graphic subject.

Sweetly, she turned the monitor for me to watch as she probed about examining the organs. After the first five minutes she said in a delighted tone, "Well, first off I'm *not* finding anything. We need to be more thorough, and take a look at your ovaries as well as above your uterus, but it's a good start."

She explained that in order to get a more accurate picture, she would need to use the new machine they'd acquired, and tried to make me laugh through the uncomfortable parts, constantly directing my attention away from my body and toward the screen.

"See—this is your left ovary . . . everything looks clean there. Why don't we take a snapshot of it so we can examine it more clearly when you're done?" And so we continued for the next twenty minutes, checking it from every angle—or at least so it seemed.

When she finished she exclaimed, "Well, you're not only clean—you're textbook perfect clean! Your organs couldn't be in better condition." She took out some of the pictures and got out a medical textbook to show me the comparison.

"See, this is a perfect uterus. Now look at your pictures. Your organs are *exactly* as they should be—perfect in size, position, proportion—perfect in every way . . . remarkable for someone your age . . . I'm going to write you a clean bill of health. We'd be happy to send your diagnosis and pictures on to your doctor— just let my nurse know the details and she'll call your doctor and send them wherever you like."

When I came back to the reception room to write my check for the examination, I was blown away by how expensive it was for that half-hour diagnostic. And yet, I've never had such a huge smile on my face when writing a check for an amount that large. I couldn't write it quickly enough. I wanted to skip out of that office!

When I walked down the hallway to the elevator, I checked to see if anyone was looking—and when the coast was clear, skipped three paces and skidded to a stop in front of the elevator door. When I stepped outside into the sunshine, I was struck once again by how beautiful L.A. seemed. Again, I was aware of how precious life seemed, and how grateful I was to be alive. And I felt a sense of awe and wonder at what an amazing miracle is stored inside the human body—how the infinite wisdom that knows how to make our hearts beat, our hair grow, that awe- some perfection of inner knowledge that secretes exactly the right amount of hormones at the right time, had worked its magic. This amazing inner power that is awake, working while we are asleep at night—what an amazing grace it is. What an awe-inspiring mystery.

It had happened just as my inner knowing had told me it would—the same part of me responsible for creating the tumor had un-created it, and I had been given the amazing gift of being allowed to participate in that process, learning what it was the tumor had to teach me.

I felt myself to be the luckiest person alive.

11

On the ride home, I felt like a horse champing at the bit—I could barely wait to get inside my house so I could call Don, who was just finishing the Mastery program in Hawaii. When I got in, I rushed to the phone, not even considering what time it might be in Hawaii, and decided to take a risk and call the front desk and see if someone could get him out of the seminar room. Sure enough, they found him in the hall, not far from the phones.

"Hello, Brandon—are you all right?" He knew it wasn't my style to call while he was in session.

"Yeah, just got back from the hospital. I've been diagnosed to be textbook perfect clean! The tumor's completely gone!"

Pause . . . as he digested just what had been said.

I began to launch into the whole story when he interrupted with, "That's incredible! You're amazing!"

By that night, word had gone out to all the trainers—not only that I had had a tumor, but that it had healed in only six weeks. When Tony heard the news, he said, quite matter-of-factly, "I knew she'd get it handled. I never thought it would be a problem for her—I really didn't. I never expected anything less."

I was glad that I had chosen to tell only people who were *certain* I could heal. They had been such a constant support, especially during those times when I began to wonder myself.

It wasn't until the next Mastery program, six months later, that I got a chance to meet up with the rest of my fellow trainers, and there were many congratulations and slaps on the back. Then once again, our hearts and minds were enthusiastically focused on the seminar, and helping the participants.

Mastery is a powerful program where speakers from all over the world, who are at the very top of their professions—real masters in their chosen fields—come together to share their knowledge and expertise with over 1,000 participants. These masters include speakers like General Norman Schwarzkopf, Dr. Deepak Chopra, Dr. John Gray, and Sir John Templeton, to name a few.

It was about half an hour before Dr. Chopra was getting ready to go on stage. I was really looking forward to hearing him—I always felt so inspired by his portion of the Mastery program because he spoke so eloquently about cellular healing and how it takes place, from a strictly scientific perspective.

He is probably the most articulate speaker on the subject of cellular healing in the field of mind-body healing today. As a highly respected endocrinologist, he took a radical approach. Instead of studying failure and the symptomology of what causes people to die, he chose to focus on success and made a life study of the process of the survivors who had healed themselves from serious disease.

I had studied with Deepak years before he'd started coming to Mastery, not having any idea how influential his work would be in supporting me on my own healing journey. I never figured that the countless case studies of people who had successfully healed themselves against the odds would end up being such a fundamental and inspirational model for me. I'd read of people with brain cancer, bone cancer—people with much more serious illnesses than I had been diagnosed with—healing themselves in record time. One woman whose entire body was riddled with cancer, who was diagnosed to die within three hours, woke up in the morning completely cancer free. So I knew if others could do it, certainly I had a good chance. It was because of their shining examples, and those of others I had helped and worked with over the years, that I had *no doubt* that my own healing journey was possible.

So on this day that Deepak got up to speak, I felt particularly grateful for both the man and his work, and I was standing in the hallway contemplating my good fortune when Tony sauntered up to me.

"Hey Brandon, why don't you get up on stage before Deepak? You've got ten minutes . . . tell everybody what happened and exactly what you did to heal yourself. You're a living example of precisely what Deepak is going to talk about—it'll be a powerful model for people. This way they can all know how to fix them-selves," he said with a good-humored smile.

On hearing that last remark I chuckled. He'd made it sound like I could just stand in front of a room and say, "Do A, then do B, then C, and you'll be 'fixed.'" Softly, not wanting to dampen his enthusiasm, and yet wanting to be firm nonetheless, I said, "You know, Tone—I'm not really willing to do that. That would be such a disservice to people. You can't say 'Do A, B and C and you'll be healed.' It's not like that. In fact *I* didn't even heal myself—the infinite intelligence inside did all the healing. I just got the incredible blessing of being allowed to *participate* in the experience. So, I wouldn't feel right getting on stage and talking about it."

Just as I finished the sentence, some other Master Trainers joined us and started playfully quipping about the previous speaker. I used that as an excuse to slip away before Tony had the chance to pursue the subject further. More than once I'd been persuaded by his powerful enthusiasm to stretch—to do some-thing I didn't really feel up to—and this was one subject that seemed somehow very sacred to me. I felt very humbled and privileged by the amazing healing journey I had undergone, deeply grateful that I'd been guided so perfectly, and I certainly didn't want to start pretending that all of a sudden I was an expert and had all the answers. More important, I didn't want people to go away thinking it was a "mind over body" thing—

because it definitely wasn't. It was a journey of discovery—surrendering, letting go, and healing. And my mind had next to nothing to do with it!

Truly, if my mind was to have figured it out, it would have done so a *long time ago*. But it hadn't, and in my process I had discovered *I needed to look someplace much deeper than the mind, to get the learning.*

How do you explain that to a group of 1,200 enthusiastic students? How do you tell people that there is a power inside all of us— an inner wisdom responsible for making our hearts beat and cells replicate, our breath go in and out even when we're asleep—and then suggest that it's possible to get in touch with that, and trust it can guide us to discover the emotional memories stored in our cells?

Then how do you explain what to *do* once you've uncovered the memories? How to completely process what was left unresolved and finally release it? How could I explain that I'd been spontaneously guided to undergo this process, and that in finally letting the emotional story go, and completely forgiving all the people involved, something unexplainable began to happen inside? That my body began to regenerate healthy cells spontaneously and automatically, without *me* having to do a thing?

How could I explain that a basketball-sized tumor can leave gracefully and cleanly in only six weeks, once the emotional pattern stored in the cells has finally been dealt with?

I walked away, thinking it was an impossible proposition, and I made sure to sequester myself completely out of sight, so that Tony wouldn't accidentally find me right before Deepak was due to go on stage. But he'd definitely got me thinking. Some part of me was saying, "Brandon, this tumor was a gift—not only to you, but to others who could benefit from what you discovered." And another part of me was saying, "Yes, but each person must undergo their own healing journey *themselves*. No one else can do it for them—it must be a *personal* journey of *discovery,* unique to each of us. Who am I to try and stand up on stage and tell people what to do? It's pure arrogance."

And so my mind battled back and forth, as I hid in the hallway, waiting for Dr. Chopra to take the stage. Once he was safely on stage, I slipped into the seminar room and stood at the back to hear his talk on cellular healing.

I'd heard it so many times before, and had always found it freshly inspiring. But this time I heard it with new ears—not as a wonderful theory, or a model of possibility, but as a statement of fact, a statement of my own experience. He was standing on stage confirming, from a scientific perspective, exactly how my tumor had left—saying it was possible to interrupt the memories stored in degenerative cells, and once the pattern was interrupted, that new healthy cells could replace them.

Having made a life's study of the successful "survivors," he said he found they had two things in common. One—they were able to get into the "Gap," get in touch with the silence of being, the infinite intelligence, the wisdom beyond the mind. Two—they were able to let go of memories stored at a cellular level.

He told the story of one woman who had been given a heart-lung transplant, and how she'd actually "inherited" the cell memories of the man who donated his organs. Upon waking up from the transplant operation, she found she had a strong craving for Chicken McNuggets and fries—even though she didn't like them! Further investigation revealed that the donor had been on his way to McDonald's to have Chicken McNuggets and fries, and had died suddenly in a motor accident.

Subsequently, she found many other memories "coming back" to her—memories of this man's family and past girlfriends, memories that had been stored in his heart and lung cells. When she met with his family privately and shared the memories that were coming up for her, they confirmed that all of the details checked out—she was literally experiencing *his* old memories as they were leaving *her* new heart cells.

Dr. Chopra explained it quite elegantly—that these "phantom memories" get passed on from one cell generation to the next. He went on to say that the cells in the various organs of the body regenerate at different speeds. The liver cells take six weeks to regenerate, whereas the skin cells take only three to four weeks. When he said that you have all new skin every three or four weeks, I remembered my last trip to Hawaii, and how, in only three weeks, my golden tan had almost completely faded away. He was right—all new skin!

He went on to say that you get a whole new stomach lining in only *four* days, and more amazing than that, all your eye cells completely replicate every *two* days. That particular scientific statistic has always seemed almost incomprehensible to me. If you're like me, you're probably asking—how is it possible that you can have all new eyeballs in only two days' time?

Then I remembered my mother's recent eye operation. On Monday she went into the hospital, and under anesthesia they slit open the front part of her eye, pulled it back, and inserted a new lens. Once the lens was in, they put the front "flap" back. Then, on Wednesday, she went back to the doctor, and he took off her eye patch. Her eye had healed perfectly, and she could see—only two days later. All new eyes in only two days.

So, I knew what Dr. Chopra was saying was not just scientific theory—it was demonstrable fact. But it still never ceases to fill me with wonder at how amazing the body's infinite intelligence is, and how quickly the body can regenerate its cells.

He then went on to ask, "If you get a whole new liver every six weeks, why is it that if you have liver cancer in January, it's still there in June? Your liver would have regenerated itself several times by then. All the cells would be entirely new." The audience sat dumbfounded by the question.

Then Dr. Chopra went on to explain that stored inside our cells are old memories—he called them "phantom memories." These old memories can eventually cause degenerative disease patterns within the cells. And before a diseased cell dies, it passes its memory onto the next cell being born. So the disease pattern continues.

He likened the human body to a computer, saying it was possible to interrupt the "programming," and that once the programming was interrupted, the possibility for healing existed. He intimated that in order to interrupt the programming, and uncover the cell memories and let them go, you would need to get in touch with the same part of you that had created the programming in the first place—the infinite intelligence, the body wisdom. And he suggested that those people who know how to get in touch with this body wisdom—to get into the "Gap," the "quantum soup," etc.—these were the successful survivors of disease.

He said it was his observation that everyone got to it in their own way, some spontaneously, some by choice—and he suggested that the possibility existed for everyone—that it was part of the quantum mechanics of the way the body healed. He confirmed in theory what had been not only my own direct personal experience but also what I had witnessed working with people over the years.

When his lecture was done, I thought about going up to him and saying, "You know, I'm exactly like all the hundreds of case studies you've documented—I underwent a similar process." But then I grew shy. I thought, "He's heard it all—it would only be old hat to him."

But I did wonder why he hadn't come up with a step-by-step process to give people. He is a medical doctor and I guess his job at the time was observing, correlating, and recording; presenting to us the overwhelming evidence that healing at a cellular level isn't simply a theory—it is proven and documented. And the benefit he was providing to humankind, through his immense research and care, is immeasurable.

When I got back from Mastery, I felt haunted by Tony's challenge. Something about it just wouldn't leave me alone. I felt so selfish—why wasn't I willing to reach out to people and share my experience with them? I realized that many people might benefit from at least being pointed in a direction that could possibly work for them.

Not only that, but alongside being a Master Trainer and seminar leader, I had been giving private one-to-ones for over ten years, serving people in letting go of all kinds of emotional issues.

I'd been trained in Neuro-Linguistic Programming, Neuro-Associative Conditioning, nutrition, kinesiology, iridology, medical hypnosis, and so many other forms of alternative therapy—and from many years of caring deeply and working closely with people I had an intuitive wisdom that served me in helping them become free. So what was holding me back? Why, when service was my life, was I keeping it to myself?

When I checked inside to see what was *really* bothering me, I wondered "How can I teach someone else how to get in touch with what Dr. Chopra calls the "Gap" or the "quantum soup"? It's not enough to *talk* about the infinite intelligence, you have to *experience* it firsthand."

For me it had been a *direct* experience. I felt it was not something you could teach to someone—*it is something your soul teaches you!* How could I explain that mystery to someone else, and more important, how could I help others connect with the deepest part of themselves and *directly* experience it? I began to wonder when I'd first spontaneously experienced this timeless awareness and whether *everyone* might have at least glimpsed it at one time or another.

Instantly, I flashed to a memory of myself at an early age. I must have been six or seven, and I remembered lying in the grass in front of my house. My mind had become completely immersed in my own private world of grass and dirt and bugs. I examined each blade of grass, noticing the tiny striated segments, and could even see the various cells in each blade. The dirt was emanating a warm, humid, earthy smell. The grass was fragrant, and I became "riveted" in my little kingdom. My mind, utterly focused, came to a complete standstill, and in that moment of absolute stillness it seemed as if time itself stood still. I found myself immersed in a bath of peace.

The grass seemed to shimmer with an intense beauty. Everything scintillated and was bursting with life. It seemed as if only a moment had gone by when I heard my mother's voice calling me in to dinner. As I got up I realized at least an hour must have slipped away as I had somehow "dropped into the Gap." My soul had quietly revealed itself to my innocent child-self.

Then my mind wandered to the various other times in my life that this vast silence of being had revealed itself to me. I realized that often the soul flashes forth at the most unexpected moments. Oddly, I flashed to a time I'd gone to see a baseball game. It was in New York City, in Yankee Stadium. Cars were lining up for miles to get in, and the fumes were noxious. It was a hot summer's day in the Bronx and tempers were flaring. I wondered, "Why am I doing this? This is crazy. All this hassle just to see a man with a bat hit a ball. No," I thought, "that's not why I go to the ballpark. There's something *special* that happens at a baseball game—something I can't explain."

I remembered getting into the stands, kids running all around, candy popcorn all over the seats, spilled Coca-Cola and sticky old beer on the floor, chewing gum on the backs of the seats. Some kid from the upper stands poured a beer over the balcony onto the guy next to me—the kid thought it was hilarious—the guy was fuming.

Then the game started, and a hush went through the audience and we stood to sing the National Anthem. A guy at the end of our row quickly broke the mood. He was drunk and began hurling obscenities at the opposing team, spilling his popcorn. Two chairs down another guy got pissed off and started yelling at him to shut up. And so the brawl began. . . . All this and the game had not yet even started!

Once again, I wondered what I was doing here, putting up with this stuff on a sweltering summer's night, and once again some inner knowing reminded me that something special happens at a ballpark—some magic would happen—I should stick it out.

And the moment came. The pitcher wound up and threw the ball; it seemed to happen in slow motion. The whole crowd became hushed as the ball approached the batter—poised, keenly alert, ready to hit the ball. Then it was as if the stadium took a breath together—one breath . . . utter stillness . . . all minds and hearts absolutely *riveted* on the ball . . . time stood still.

Then—WHACK! The bat sending the ball soaring into the outfield . . . hair standing on end, ripples of ecstasy and joy flowing all over, pealing with laughter, cheering for joy . . . *Magic!*

A simple but common moment in a normal everyday sports game. But what had made it so magical—a ball hitting a bat? I don't think so. What was it about that moment that made it so special?

I played the whole scene over again in my head, only this time I slowed it down. Ball comes . . . everyone and everything stops . . . *mind comes to complete standstill*, and in that gap of absolute silence the soul flashes forth—an immensity revealing itself . . . a presence of vastness . . . a greatness that can't be explained . . . and then *whack!*—ball hit, hair standing on end. Something great had revealed itself in that tiny instant. One heart, one breath, hair on end. We'd dropped into the "Gap" for an instant and this vast truth had, in a flash, revealed itself.

No wonder we love to go to sports events. All of us have probably been to a basketball or football game and had the experience when it seemed as if for a moment everything came to a standstill while the crowd was held in suspense and, for an instant, an unexplainable energy arose from inside, making our hair stand on end? Isn't it true we secretly wait for that "magic moment"? We know it may only happen for one tiny instant, but it'll be worth putting up with all the rest of it.

Then my mind flashed to another experience of Source, to my first honeymoon night with Don. We'd bought tickets to see Rudolf Nureyev in the ballet *Romeo and Juliet* at the Metropolitan Opera House. At that time Nureyev was already a legend and he was at his absolute peak.

Once again, there was a moment where it seemed as if time stood still. It was as if Nureyev reached into the depths of his soul—into genius itself. He leaped into the air, and his legs spread into a full split; then, for a moment, it was as if he lifted even higher—as if he was practically floating in the air. Once again the whole audience drew a breath, one heart, hair on end.

Ripples of cause-less joy spread through the theatre. It was as if in the moment Nureyev tapped into his inner genius, the same thing in all of us instantly recognized itself. Our own greatness flashed forth. We'd seen our Selves in the mirror. No way to explain it, but it had been undeniable, palpable. Everyone got it at the same time. "Self"-recognition.

When Nureyev came out for his bows we all just leaped to our feet. Tears streaming, hands clapping, clapping, clapping. We couldn't thank the man enough. We kept him coming back for forty-three minutes of a huge outpouring of cheering and ovations. I know because we missed our dinner reservation! My hands were purple, and yet I couldn't stop applauding. I was so grateful to this man for tapping into his soul, and mainly I was thankful that the genius inside *me* had remembered itself.

Have you ever had that experience at the end of an exceptional play or concert where you felt yourself swept along by the beauty of the music, and your sense of separate self dropped away? Or perhaps you've had that experience in nature? Have you ever stood on a mountaintop, awed by the vastness? Or found your being hushed by the beauty of a sunset by the sea? Or perhaps you've had the experience of skiing "out of your mind," feeling like a river flowing down the slopes—completely at one with the mountain and lost in a grace that intrinsically "knew" how and when to turn.

All of us *must* have had this kind of experience at one point in our lives. Perhaps you've had the experience of being swept along by the flowing rhythm of the music while dancing and found your mind was no longer directing your feet—that they seemed to have a life of their own.

I realized that there were so many times I'd dropped into "Source" spontaneously. Yet the challenge still lay before me— how to help others have a direct *sustained* experience of this?

The soul had chosen such times to reveal its boundless expansion, but how to tap into that by *choice*, and then how to help someone else remain in a *sustained* experience of it long enough to be able to go through a healing process? How to help someone *directly* experience this boundlessness, this peace, this eternal love? How to help someone discover for themselves that this has always been and would always be *who they really are?* That it is who they are in their essence, in the very core of their being? And that as soon as the mind gets out of its own way the "real" Self would be revealed?

How to help someone realize that there is no need to turn to anyone or anything *outside?* That this power, this consciousness, this presence of love, this oneness that is whole, silent, and keenly aware, call it what you will—*is your own true nature!* How could I assist someone in discovering something that only *they* can discover and directly experience *personally?*

I knew that no amount of words could capture it, that the best that words could do was *point* at it, but that the experience of it could come only from *experience* itself, from the boundless greatness revealing itself.

I thought, "Everyone *must* have glimpsed this truth at some point or another in their life—surely." Their minds *had* to have been arrested at some point or another. How could you have watched Torvill and Dean skating to *Bolero* on their way to Olympic gold and not had a moment of riveted stillness, absolute awe, when the inner genius revealed itself?

Perhaps *you* may have heard John F. Kennedy proclaim, "Ask not what your country can do for you, ask what you can do for your country" or Martin Luther King exclaim, "I have a dream . . ." or Neil Armstrong transmit from the moon, "That's one small step for a man, one giant leap for mankind." Moments when truth itself spoke and then truth inside you recognized itself.

So often when someone taps into that inner genius, into the truth, something inside us stirs—the hair stands on end, and an inner "yes" is felt. Truth recognizing itself. But how to get truth to recognize itself by *choice?*

So I stopped giving one-on-ones for a while. Until I could find a way to give someone a *sustained* experience of their *true self*, I felt I wouldn't be serving people at their deepest level. And I knew it is when the emotional issues are addressed at the *deepest* level—at the level of the soul, of consciousness itself—that you really get to the *core* of the issue. It's then that *true freedom*, emotionally as well as physically, can take place. Then *real* healing begins.

Mine had been a spiritual journey—one of letting go into freedom. The *result* had been healing at a very physical, cellular level. The evidence was unmistakable, and yet I couldn't touch or test, or even explain, the unexplainable power and mystery of the soul.

So the prayer continued to go out—I wanted to be guided to find a way to help others experience it themselves. I wanted to assist them in healing on *all* levels—not just the physical, but also the emotional and spiritual.

As I didn't have the answers I thought it best to continue my own personal spiritual journey and put my quest to help others have a sustained experience of Source on the back burner. I decided to trust that if I was meant to help others, somehow a way would be revealed.

Several months later, when I least expected it, the answer was profoundly revealed. I was given a direct experience of Source so enormous that the full realization of it has not left me since that day. **Source has been present as the undercurrent of my life ever since.**

12

I was taking a course with a spiritual teacher when, during a question and answer session, one of the students asked, "What do I do if an intense emotion comes up for me—how do I find the peace in that?"

She answered, "Just *don't move*. Let yourself be completely present to the emotion. Welcome it. If a negative emotion arises, don't run away from it; don't run off to the refrigerator to eat some food to cover it up; don't turn on the television to distract yourself from it; don't call your friends to disperse its energy by gossiping about it. Just stop and *feel* it. Just let yourself *be present* to it. You'll find if you don't try to distract yourself from it, or push it away, or, worse still, dump it on someone else; if you *stay still,* if you are really *present* to it—in the very core of the feeling you will find peace. So when you feel a powerful emotion, just let it be—DON'T MOVE. *Welcome it*."

I thought, "What a radical idea." Everything in the self-help movement is teaching us to change our thoughts, make them more positive. Or if you don't change your thoughts, then change your physiology—do anything you can to *avoid* the pain. Even see a medical doctors who'll prescribe drugs to dull the emotional intensity. "Act as if"—do whatever you can to make sure you *don't* allow yourself to *really feel* what's coming up. She was saying something totally different—"Don't move. Be present." What a novel concept!

Something inside me stirred. I said to myself, "What if she's right? What if, instead of 'reframing' my emotions, I simply welcomed them and allowed them to be *fully felt?* I wonder if I might find this peace she is speaking about in the core of the feeling?"

So I decided to give it a try. What did I have to lose? That had always been my way: I could never take anything at face value—I always had to *experience* what someone was talking about before I could take it on board.

I knew I had a long-standing emotional issue that I needed to look at and resolve. I had been compelled by a need to help and serve others—even when it cost me my health. I just didn't know how to say no. So I thought this might be the perfect opportunity to investigate what she meant.

Don was going to be away giving seminars for five days. Why didn't I use that time to really check her theory out? So before Don left, I let him know that I was going to try an experiment. I was going to take the five days and go into silence, and instead of using all the old techniques, I was going to do what the spiritual teacher had suggested—go right into the heart of the emotional feeling and discover what was at the *core* of it.

I explained to him that she had suggested that you do not distract yourself from the emotion, gossiping about it or going to the movies to get away from it or eating or watching TV to avoid it—that you should just allow yourself to really *feel* it. So, I didn't know what would happen, but I really felt pulled to give it a try.

I asked him not to phone me as I didn't want to use that as an excuse to distract myself. I really wanted to give it my all. He and I had both been on several silent spiritual retreats before, so it was nothing new to him, and he was glad to give me the support.

As he was departing, Don said, "I'll miss you—I really love our nightly phone calls—I'll miss the contact. You know, Brandon, I'm always saying to my students at the seminars, 'I go away for a weekend and I never know who I'm going to come back to!' You're always growing so much."

I replied lightly, "No one could say it ever gets boring or stale around here."

"No . . . no chance of that!"

He wished me luck, and I could feel that inwardly he admired my perseverance. As he was going out the door, I kissed him goodbye, and somehow it didn't feel like our usual soft, romantic parting. It felt like a sad, almost longing farewell—as if he were off on a long ocean voyage, and I'd been left on an island, marooned, unable to reach him.

"What nonsense," I said to myself, trying to shake the feeling off. As I shut the door, I began to notice a sick sensation growing in the pit of my stomach, as if something *big* was about to happen. A shiver went through me as a strong sense of foreboding washed over me.

Again I tried to shake it off as I ran over to the balcony to wave my usual goodbye. As the car pulled off, I strode back into the living room, chastising myself inwardly—"This is ridiculous—he's only going away for five days . . . pull yourself together."

Mentally, I pulled myself up by the bootstraps, and half marched myself into the kitchen to make a little salad for lunch. While preparing it, I was aware that part of me was trying to keep myself busy, to distract myself from the growing sense of foreboding. As I chopped the salad and minced the vegetables, I could feel a subtle, but very present fear lurking in the background. The salad seemed particularly unsatisfying, and I sat and ate a very unsettled, restless meal.

During lunch, I got the notion that I should probably prepare myself for the "big experiment" by making sure the house was cleaned, the laundry done, and the bills paid and in the mail. Some part of me knew this was an avoidance tactic, to prolong the period of time before I had to face the emotional issue, and part of me felt it was probably a good idea to "clear the decks" so that I wouldn't have any distractions.

I busied myself putting everything in order, making some last-minute phone calls to alert my daughter and friends that I was taking time off, and then I finished it all by changing the announcement on the answering machine: "Hi, there—you've reached Don and Brandon. Don will be out of town for five days, and I'll be on a silent retreat, so we won't be able to get back to you until Monday. We look forward to speaking to you then. Please leave a message at the sound of the beep."

It sounded so final—like I'd cut myself off from all communication with the world. I reached to turn the volume control all the way down, and something inside stopped me. I thought, "Even if I won't be speaking to them, at least I can hear their voices."

At this last thought, I laughed inwardly at how dramatic I was making all of this seem. I reminded myself how much I had enjoyed taking silent time in the past, and tried to convince myself that this time was no different. But my body wasn't believing the words. It felt like my mind was trying to give me a snow job, and I just wasn't buying it.

With no more chores to distract me, I became all too aware of the sick feeling of fear building inside. I strode down the stairs into the living room, and decided the time had come—I would finally face this emotional issue. I sat down in our big, soft, peach-colored chair and thought, "Now what?"

As I sat there, I became aware that something inside seemed to be *driving* me to be of service to anyone and everyone who came into my life. I would help someone no matter what time of day or night, so much so that I had often completely ignored my own needs, and definitely had burned myself out more than once, working continuously day and night for sometimes weeks on end.

It was when I was giving to others, and helping them in some way, that I felt my best. In the seminars with Tony I would often get only a few hours' sleep, and yet I would thrive on it—feeling I was really giving my all. But I could also see that it had moved well beyond healthful and enthusiastic support into an unhealthy *need* to be of service. It was as if my whole identity had become tied up in selfless service.

I recalled one incident that really drove home to me the depth to which it was running my life. Two years before, after enjoying twelve years of absolutely vibrant health, my body gave me a "wake up or else!" warning. It came directly after a fourteen-day program with Tony during which I had taken on so many jobs that I was getting only two or three hours' sleep per night. Some nights I only got a shower, changed clothes, then went back to work.

At the end of it, I felt emotionally, deeply fulfilled, very rewarded—feeling my efforts had made a huge difference in a lot of people's lives. But my body felt differently. It said, "Stop. Enough!"—and I ended up in bed with acute pneumonia.

Every health professional I went to at that time said exactly the same thing to me—"Brandon, you have suppressed exhaustion buried in your cells. You're just going to have to wait this one out, and take rest and heal. How do you plan to be around to help others if you aren't willing to take care of yourself? If you don't stop, your body will stop you."

I listened to what they said, and made the decision that I couldn't afford *not* to heed their advice. So, little by little, over the next two years, I began to learn how to look out for myself and create more balance in my life. It was hard though, because whenever I did take time out just for myself, I felt guilty and secretly ashamed—like I should be out there helping and serving.

The love of service had definitely become a *need,* an *addiction,* an *obsession.* My identity had become tied up in the noble, selfless image I held of myself. So, as I sat down in that peach chair, I knew I wasn't sitting there to face and resolve just any old emotional issue. I was there to face one of the biggest issues of my life—to examine my very identity, to find out what was driving me, and more than that, to find out what was at the core of it all.

It didn't feel like a small thing. It felt huge. And as I sat there, innocent and open, I didn't know where to begin. I felt very alone. I didn't have a teacher to point the way and help me through. My husband wasn't there to hold my hand. I was completely on my own. Silently I made a strong vow not to distract myself from the project—not to make any phone calls to reach out to people—nor would I receive any either. I wasn't going to indulge this addiction—not for five days. I was simply going to do what the teacher said: "In the face of emotion, don't move, welcome it."

So I sat in the chair. After about five minutes I began to sweat. My heart began to pound at the very thought that I wouldn't be allowing myself to get up and answer the phone to anyone needing help. My mind began to race to all the people in my life that I "should" be reaching out to. So, to calm my mind, I decided I'd start the big experiment with meditation.

But even that was difficult, as it brought the fear more fiercely into my face. The question arose, "If I'm not serving anyone, and there's no service to be done, and no one serving—then who am I?"

There was an inner scrambling, an overwhelming fear that if there was no service being done, and no one doing the service, then *there would be no one there*. I decided to let myself face the fear straight on—not to run away from it, but just allow myself to feel it completely, be overwhelmed by it if need be—but stick to the teacher's advice—"Welcome it, and don't move."

So I sat there holding the sides of the chair, and allowed myself to feel the full energy of the fear. My hands were sweating, and my body felt flooded by it. As I welcomed this fear I began sinking inwardly. I sank into a loneliness—a loneliness so deep it seemed as if the whole room was lonely. It felt like the chairs emanated loneliness, and the walls were lonely; a loneliness so profound, all the molecules in the room vibrated with it. It seemed there was no place the loneliness was not, and still I kept my vow. No matter what the emotion, I would *not* move—I would just be present to it, feel it completely, and let myself be carried into the very core of it. I had never known such loneliness, and didn't know how painful it could be, but still I didn't move.

After some time, I began sinking from loneliness into another "layer" of emotion. I fell into a despair so deep I didn't know I could feel that hopeless. It was the feeling, "If there's no service being given, and no one to serve, then what's the use of living; why bother?"

There was a feeling of just giving up, and a willingness to pack it all in—to die. I'd never experienced such overwhelming pain mixed so completely with utter hopelessness and helplessness. Despair was everywhere, and there was no avoiding it.

Just when it seemed as if the despair would overwhelm me, I felt myself sinking again through yet another layer, only this time I seemed to be standing on the edge of what appeared to be an abyss—a black hole, an absolute nothingness. Terror arose as a sickly cold sweat broke out all over my body. I felt that I would die if I went in "there."

I froze. I got absolutely stuck and resistant. If I had to go into that blackness of annihilation, I wasn't willing to continue—no matter what the teacher had said. So I just stood there, in my mind's eye, frozen on the edge of what I was certain would be my own death—or at least the death of Brandon as I knew her.

The terror was overwhelming; tears flashed from my eyes, my hands gripped the chair. I just couldn't face whatever was in that black void of nothingness.

After a time, the terror made me feel exhausted, and yet I still kept my commitment. *I would not move.* I was stuck, unable and unwilling to surrender into that black hole, yet unwilling to go back on my vow. I was frozen in terror, and didn't know what to do.

Still I didn't move. Time went by. Finally a question arose— "What if I were *never* to leave this place, and I were stuck here always?" And in that moment, something happened. It was as if my will finally caved in, and I surrendered. I found myself free-falling . . . free-falling through nothingness, and expanding into a peace that mere words can't begin to describe.

The entire room filled with peace. It radiated peace. I was peace, and I was also everything in the room. Peace and an indescribable love seemed to fill the room. I was the love that is the source of life itself. I was the molecules dancing, and all the spaces in between.

Everything in the room seemed to scintillate with shining peace, and yet simultaneously I had the profound, undeniable recognition that this peace was not a passing state, nor was it something outside me. It *was* me. I'd fallen into my very soul. And my soul was everything. I felt boundless, limitless, eternal, timeless—I felt as if this that I am reached beyond the reaches of the universe, with all of life happening *in* me.

I realized that this must be the "peace that passeth all understanding"—the peace *beyond* understanding, beyond the comprehension of the mind. *I knew myself as pure awareness, absolute freedom, limitless love.*

I was reminded of the words of the great Sufi poet, Kabir:

The way of love is not
A subtle argument.
The door there is devastation.
Birds make great sky-circles of their freedom.
How do they learn it?
They fall, and falling,
They're given wings.

This love, this freedom, has been with me, *as me*, ever since that moment. I know it to be who I am; not a passing state, but *who I am at my core.* This is the *only* real truth. This is "Home." It had happened exactly as the spiritual teacher had said it would. Right in the very core of *any* feeling is peace itself. Peace with a capital *P*. Ultimate Peace.

Spontaneously, I had dropped through the limiting emotional layers that seemed to obscure me from knowing my true self, my soul. These layers had become like veils that had kept my true self hidden from me. All I'd done was peel one veil, one layer back at a time. It was like peeling the layers of an onion, only what I'd found in the core was a diamond of flawless perfection, of indescribable beauty. I'd unearthed a shining brilliance that no words can describe.

It reminded me of the story at the beginning of this book, only now it wasn't only a pretty metaphor, it was my own experience. I'd heard it said that when we are born, we come in as a pristine, pure, flawless diamond, and through the course of life we dump a lot of emotional "shit" on top of it, and obscure its natural brilliance and radiance. Then, when we become adults, we paint varnish over it, to make it all appear shiny and presentable. All we've really done is put a hard polished veneer over a bunch of crap. When we present it to the world saying, "This is who I am," we wonder why it is no one buys it.

Then one day, if we're very lucky, through some act of grace, or through a transformative seminar, a book, a crisis, a disease, or some other gift of life, we might have the great good fortune to break through and crack this brittle surface. Then for a while it might seem as if all we're doing is shoveling through the brown stuff. But eventually, underneath it all, we unearth the priceless diamond that has always been there—shining, pristine, pure and exquisitely beautiful.

We eventually realize that we've *always* been this flawless diamond, only we'd spent the whole of our lives thinking we were the stuff that obscured it. For some of us, even though we'd glimpsed our own inner radiance, it wouldn't take long before we'd forget it, or ignore it, and once again we'd identify with our polished, artificial surfaces.

This story had finally revealed its true meaning for me. I'd dropped through the layers of my rubbish, and had spontaneously discovered the flawless diamond—a realization that *no one* could take from me. No emotion could make it go away, no life experience could stain it, no criticism could mar it, for it is by nature unstained, pristine, and untouched by the whole of life's drama. It's who I am, who you are, and who we always will be. I came to realize that the whole world had come alive, and was scintillating and *sparkling as me*.

I continued to stay in silence for the full five days, but now I no longer felt the need to call friends and clients to offer my services. Nor did I feel compelled to pick up the phone at the first request for help. I no longer needed to serve in order to get love and appreciation. Why would I seek love from others when I'd realized *I am love?*

What an irony! I had spent a lifetime earning others' love, approval, and admiration by giving, serving, helping, caring, and striving to do my best, even if it meant sacrificing my own needs and personal desires or goals, and *even* if it destroyed my health. And here I'd discovered that this love and self-worth I'd been seeking had been there all along! Nothing to do to get it—just *be* it, know it.

So, basking in my own love, I was happy to peacefully go about my daily household chores. Not because they would give me anything, or prove that I was a good person, but just because they were natural things to do. Effortless Being.

Since that experience, I've found myself resting in this effortless being. I no longer feel compelled or driven to do, do, do to help every person I know. The difference is that I'm no longer *driven* by the need to get love, to be worthy, to get approval. Service takes place as a natural aspect of my life, simply because it's the natural expression of the love that is always there. It is born out of an easy flow of love, and it feels to me as if all of my life is taking place in this "flow."

Most surprising of all, I found it became as easy to *receive* love as to give it. This was a real revelation for me. In the past I'd always been the caregiver, the strong one—I'd created an entire identity around being there in support and service. I would have felt ashamed, an absolute failure, if I had to ask for help or guidance, or needed emotional support. Even to receive material gifts from loved ones was difficult for me. I was much more comfortable in the serving role.

In the presence of real love it doesn't matter whether I'm giving or receiving—it just seems to flow through, and it's beautiful no matter which direction it comes from. More accurately, it doesn't even feel like giving and receiving—just action taking place in a vast presence of love.

Now I'm finally willing to admit I need help, that I don't have all the answers. I'm finally willing to be real with my loved ones—not *acting* strong but *being* strong enough to realize I can't do it all on my own—that I genuinely need help, and I feel so humbly grateful for the support and guidance of others.

So many lessons have come out of that one experiment and the lessons keep coming daily. However, the task still lay before me. Now that I'd experienced it myself, how to translate all that into a practical, step-by-step plan or map so that others could go on their own personal journey of unlayering and Self-discovery? And then, once they had uncovered the boundless love, the vast silence of the soul, how to help them discover the memories stored in the cells?

Then, once the cell memories were uncovered, how to help them *resolve* and heal the old unresolved issues? Then how to assist them in *finishing* their old painful stories? Finally, once that was completed, how to teach them to trust that the body would know how to heal itself naturally, automatically, of its own accord, without them having to do anything to "make" it happen?

How to teach people that this is a process of participation with the soul, and once old patterns, issues, and memories are healed, that the body intrinsically knows how to do the rest? How to assist people in learning to *trust,* and help them to move from "doer-ship" to "be-er-ship"?

I realized this was no small task. Yet I also knew that I'd been given a key—a key to falling into the "Gap," to getting in touch with the truth. *I'd found a way to have a sustained direct experience of the infinite intelligence, Source.* Now the question was, just because it worked for me, did that mean it would necessarily work for others? So I decided to find out.

13

I put out a prayer that people who felt "hooked" by a challenging emotional issue would somehow be guided to work with me. I specifically put out the intention to work with people who felt they had no hope—people who had tried everything to heal from an emotional issue; people who, like me, had done all kinds of seminars; people who had done a huge amount of introspection, or gone through years of therapy; people who, even though they had tried and tried, were still haunted by their old issue—as if it was running on automatic pilot.

I had been completely hooked by the need to serve others, and it had been controlling my life. By going down through the emotional layers I had become free. So I wanted to draw to me those who, like me, really wanted to be free and were willing to roll up their sleeves and get down to work.

I knew that we *all* have issues we're hooked by. There are only so many negative emotions, and we've all had them come up at some time or another. I thought of some of the more common ones—anger, rage, frustration, anxiety, loss, depression, betrayal, feeling inferior or unworthy, low self-esteem, jealousy, sadness or hurt, sensitivity to criticism, loneliness, abandonment, grief, despair, fear of the loss of a loved one, fear of failure or judgment, and so on.

I knew these were the emotional issues we all get trapped by, and I thought that if we were all capable of dropping through the emotional layers, as I had done, and if we were *all* capable of discovering our true selves, beyond the pain—what an amazing gift that would be. What if we could all pull back the layers of the onion to reveal the love and peace that is at our core?

As I had never done the process with anyone but myself, I wanted to start by working with my closest friends and loved ones. The next day I received a phone call from my friend Nancy. During our conversation she suggested that it could be fun to give seminars together. I had told her that I might be open to the idea, but that I wasn't really interested in doing any of the material I'd done in the past. I wanted to do work that was born out of my most current realizations and transformations, but I wasn't completely clear yet what it was I had to teach; I was only clear that I'd undergone a powerful healing journey that could be of benefit to other people in pointing them onto their own journeys.

Later on in the conversation, she alluded to some emotional problems that she and her husband, Ronald, were having. So I said to Nancy, "Why don't we try a recent process I underwent, and see where it takes us? Unlike me, you'll actually have someone by your side to see you through it, and I'll be able to help if there are any scary parts. As I've gone through it myself, I bet I'll be able to help you through it more quickly. Working at the level of the soul is definitely what my heart feels called to do. I can't guarantee it will work, because I haven't tried it with anyone else, but I'm willing to go for it if you are."

Nancy agreed, and said that she could barely wait to roll up her sleeves and finally go after this issue. So we made an appointment for the next morning. As I put down the phone I thought that I would probably have to call on all of my expertise in the field of NLP, and I trusted that the wisdom born of years of transformational work would likely be of service to her in her process. And though my own process had been long, painful, and arduous seeming, I figured that, now I understood the unlayering principle, there were probably some linguistic tools I could use to help her go through her emotional layers more quickly and easily than I had done.

The next day, we met at Nancy's place. As we sat down on the soft carpeting in her bedroom, I asked her if she would mind if we put out a prayer for guidance, as this was the first time I would be trying the process with someone else. She replied that she felt touched that I cared so much to want to help her in the first place. Recently she had felt emotionally incapacitated by a jealous rage that kept arising. No matter what she told herself to soften the feeling, some part of her was just not buying it, and the rage seemed to come spontaneously, out of nowhere. She knew it was irrational, and there was no basis for it in her husband's actions, but she just couldn't seem to stop it from blowing up. She was newly married, and feared that if the jealousy didn't stop, she might lose her husband.

She said she was willing to try anything at this point. She just wanted to find out why this was happening, and become free from it. She kept assuring me that this just wasn't like her. She'd not known such jealousy in the past, and she didn't know where it was coming from right now.

Assuring her that I was happy to assist her in any way I knew how, I felt I also had to tell her I just couldn't give her any guarantees. I'd been set free spontaneously from my issue of needing to serve by following the words of a spiritual teacher. I didn't know if she would undergo the same unlayering process, nor if she would get the same result, but I was willing to give it a try.

She knew my extensive background as a therapist and a seminar leader, and she said, "Brandon, you've had such a profound effect on so many people's lives. I'm really open to trying anything you feel might help. Let's just go for it." Her enthusiasm and openness were heartening, and inspired me freshly to give it my all. So together we sat silently and prayed. I made a special prayer that she'd truly become free. I had spoken to her husband and he'd asked me to do what I could to help, as he couldn't face any more of her irrational-seeming outbursts. He'd gone into shutdown mode himself, and he feared that he might have reached the limit—he was near "threshold" with it all.

I really wanted to help them both. And so we began. I asked her just to sit, be present, and allow herself to fully *feel* the jealousy—to really allow it to come up. She chuckled, "No problem there," as the emotion erupted, and her face became bright pink. I asked her where in her body she felt the jealousy most strongly. She pointed to her chest. I could see that the feeling was very intense for her, so I quickly asked her what was behind it or underneath it.

Unexpectedly, she spontaneously sank through to the next emotional layer—anger. Once again I reminded her to let the feeling be *fully* experienced, to be present to it. Her face turned red and her body began to shake. She said, "It's not really anger, it's rage."

"Well, go ahead and just allow yourself to *really feel* this rage."

Her body tensed as she allowed it all to come up and be fully felt.

"Now I wonder what's behind it, what's underneath it? Just allow yourself to drop through." I could see her sinking through to the next emotion.

"Hurt," she said, as tears flashed to her eyes.

"Where in your body do you feel this hurt?" I asked.

"Here, in my solar plexus."

She began to cry openly, and as I could see that she was fully welcoming the feeling, I gently asked her once again, "What's beneath that?"

Once again she fell through to another layer—"Abandonment."

Before I could ask her where in her body she felt this feeling, she said, "Is it okay to talk?"

"Sure," I said, not knowing if it might be a distraction. She'd done so well up until now, being present and fully feeling the feelings, and I knew it was essential for her to just stay with the raw, pure emotion, and not distract herself or avoid it.

I was getting ready to make sure she got back on track, and just stayed in the pure emotion, when she blurted out, "I see a memory of when I was eight years old. My sister, my best girlfriend, and I were playing on the beach. Then my sister ran off to play with my best girlfriend, and I felt totally abandoned, lost, as if she'd stolen away all the love and friendship in my life."

I was busy writing down everything she said, and I thought— "We'll get to this later. Right now she still needs to keep 'peeling back the layers of this onion.' " I said, "Thank you. I wrote it all down; we'll get to it later. Let's stick with the pure emotion that you're feeling—so just feel that pure abandonment. . . . What's beneath that?"

Her posture visibly changed, and she said, "I feel so lost, so alone."

"Then feel that fully. Be present to it," I said.

Her face filled with a forlorn look that made her appear lost and childlike. Then there was a long pause as her face grew pale. Then she muttered breathily, "Oh, shit. I've sunk into something I've never seen before. There's this black hole here; it's like a void."

I thought, "I know this place all too well—she's there! I hope she'll have the courage to dive in." It had been such a stopping place for me, and I prayed that somehow I'd be able to reassure her enough to get her to relax into it. I said gently, "Well, just let yourself go into it."

She replied, "I can't. I'm scared."

"Scared is okay. Just let yourself fall right into the nothingness." She began to shake, and then her breath stopped for a moment. Inwardly I felt a tinge of panic, and then I watched as a deep relaxation spread all over her body, and a little smile began to play across her face.

"So what are you feeling?" I asked, really curious by this time.

"Laughter!"—as she began to laugh out loud. "What was I afraid of?"

"Where do you feel that?"

"In my belly, but kind of all over," she replied, as she shook with laughter.

"Great, now what's beyond even this?"

"I feel childlike, playful, happiness all over."

"Great! Feel it fully," I said.

She began to glow. "Now what's beyond even that?"

"JOY!" Her emotion seemed contagious. It felt so pervasive, I caught it myself. "I feel like I'm just radiating joy, like it's everywhere," she enthused.

Something inside me still felt that she wasn't quite there yet, so I asked once more, "What's beyond that?"

And then a great presence of peace filled the room as she grew absolutely still. A look of peace and awe radiated from her face.

"Eternal. It's eternal . . . I'm everything . . . I'm everywhere . . . It's God . . . Bliss. There are no words, Brandon."

"I know," I thought. "There are no words."

She'd done it! She realized herself to be the same boundless awareness for which there are no words. And, instead of taking hours, she'd taken only minutes!

"Beautiful . . ." I said to her. "Beautiful. Just rest in this, *as this*."

I was stunned and awed. We'd taken only about fifteen minutes. Yet she was clearly having a profound experience of her own essence, her true self. As I sat there with her, I too felt that immense peace, as if I'd gone through the layers with her. And so, for a while, we just sat together drinking in the indescribable beauty of truth.

"Now what?" I wondered. "How can I bring this peace into the healing process so that she can have access to the wisdom that arises naturally from it?"

Even though her experience of her own Source was profound, I knew it wasn't enough just to leave her in the presence of it. She still had to process the memory that had spontaneously come up. I knew that the reason my tumor had left was not just because I knew how to access my soul, but because I'd found the issue that was stored in my body, and finally resolved it and finished the story—*it was a combination of both*. Even though the vast, boundless, eternal Self is in and of itself immense, it still isn't the whole picture.

How could we get the wisdom born of this vast, boundless

peace to speak to the various emotional layers she'd gone through, and more important, bring it directly to the memory itself? So I decided very simply to ask her to speak from this place of peace to the various emotional layers. "If this vast eternalness, this peace, this love, had something to say to the previous emotional layer, joy, what would it say?" I asked.

When she began to speak, I put my pen down, riveted by the wisdom pouring from her. She said, "I *am* joy! Joy is always at my very core. I only need to turn my attention to it, and it's always there."

I had never heard Nancy speak so simply and beautifully before. It seemed as if truth was speaking. So I asked the same question with the next layer up, and once again, what she said was so inspired it brought tears to my eyes. And so, in the same way, we continued, letting her own inner wisdom speak to each layer.

I sat humbled, as it seemed that truth was not just speaking the wisdom, but that it seemed to be dissolving all the pain of her previous emotional layers. It was as if the words springing from Nancy's mouth were an antidote to the pain she had experienced. When she finished speaking to each layer, it was as if the pain that had been there dissolved in the vast energy and peace that was in the room.

When she got up to the abandonment layer I looked down at my sheet, and noticed that that was the point at which the memory had appeared. I thought, "As it seems that the soul knows perfectly and precisely how to run this whole process, I'm sure the memory came at this level for a reason and a purpose. It seems like now would be the right time to address her old memory—to take Nancy through the same healing process I'd gone through with my tumor."

So, remembering my experience with Surja, I asked her to imagine a campfire, and to put the various people who were in her memory by the fire. I suggested that she also bring to the campfire a mentor whose wisdom she trusted, and in whose presence she felt safe. And so her fireside chat began.

Her process went much as mine had gone, and as the younger

Nancy spoke to her sister and her best friend of the abandonment and hurt she had felt, it seemed as if years of unspoken, unexpressed pain were finally being expressed and leaving. Then she listened as her sister and her best friend shared what they were going through at the time. Nancy seemed genuinely surprised to hear that it was not her sister's intent to steal her best friend away—that they were just running off to have some fun. Nancy's sister apologized sincerely for the pain that had come out of their actions.

When it seemed as if they'd finally resolved the whole issue, I asked Nancy if she felt complete—was there anything still unspoken that she needed to share with her sister? She replied that she wanted to thank her sister, that she'd never known how she'd felt, and she wanted her to know that, even though they'd had a lot of misunderstandings through the years, she loved her. Then I asked her again if she felt she was completely empty; had she said everything she needed to say, and heard everything she needed to hear?

She replied simply, "Yeah."

Remembering how important forgiveness had been in my own process, I asked Nancy if she was finally willing to completely forgive her sister, from the bottom of her heart.

Quietly, she answered, "Yes."

Tears streamed down her cheeks as she finally forgave her sister for a betrayal she'd held on to for years—a betrayal that had, in fact, *never actually occurred,* except in the younger Nancy's mind.

"Hmm," I thought, "it's uncanny how similar this is to what is happening right now in her life. She's feeling betrayed by Ronald, her husband, and has an unexplainable jealousy and rage for something that *hasn't even occurred.*"

It's amazing to me how we store inside these old emotional patterns, which play themselves out again and again only with different people. Same issue, just different players! And yet we never seem to resolve the pain or learn the lessons; we just keep running the same old pattern over and over again!

A friend of mine had once come to me complaining that she just seemed to go from one relationship to another. She'd said it was as if she just packed all her bad habits, old wounded patterns and emotional baggage into a suitcase. Then she'd get into the next relationship, open the suitcase, and the same old emotional patterns would play themselves out. Then she'd pack them all up again, leave the relationship and go on to the next, open the suitcase, get all her emotional baggage out . . . And so it would go, over and again. She said she was tired of never learning her lessons, but instead just re-running the old habits.

Nancy reminded me of this friend. Here Nancy was, running her childhood abandonment issue and the jealousy that came out of it, with her husband Ronald. If she didn't wake up to it soon, she might actually create what she most feared—that her irrational jealousy would drive him away, and he would, in fact, abandon her. Then she'd finally have a real, not imagined, reason to feel abandoned.

I thought, "We all do this. Isn't it amazing that we aren't given a manual when we are born telling us what to do about all of this, and how to handle it when these things come up?"

When the memory processing was finished, I asked Nancy to once again let her own inner wisdom speak to the remaining levels, and let the energy of peace dissolve any remaining pain. When she was finished, I did what's known as a "future integration" (a standard NLP means of checking with the other-than-conscious mind to make sure the processing is all integrated). I asked her to look into the future one day from now, one week from now, one month, six months, one year . . . and so on, to see how at each juncture she was handling her old abandonment/jealousy issue.

As Nancy looked one day into the future, she said she definitely felt easier, lighter—like it wasn't much of an issue, but that she would have to consciously be aware *not* to imagine that her husband might be doing something behind her back. At one week it was easier still to let go of the old pattern, but she occasionally had to remind herself. At one month it was hardly an issue at all, and at six months it never even came up for her again. At one year she felt herself free and joyous, and at five years she was blown away by the wisdom and freedom she developed. Ten years down the line, she said she felt like she was light, radiance, and joy itself.

Figuring that the "future her" was pretty wise, I said, "Why don't you let the wisdom of the future you give the present-day you some advice? Why don't you write a letter from the future you giving the present you some practical advice on what to do, what to say, what to think, how to be, what kinds of actions to take, how to help your relationship with Ronald, and so on?"

When she opened her eyes, I handed her a piece of paper, upon which she promptly began to write a letter to herself. She wrote for some time, and when she was done, she put her pen down, and with a laugh said, "The future me had a lot to say— and not just about Ronald, but about a lot of things in my life."

Handing me the letter, she said, "What do you think?" I read it, once again thinking, "This is the wisdom of the ages; this is like modern western sutras. It really is not only profound, but extremely practical." I thanked her for sharing it with me, and suggested that she put it up on her bathroom mirror to remind her of the various commitments she had made to herself.

Three days later, when I caught up with Nancy, she said the jealousy issue wasn't coming up for her anymore. Delighted, I still wasn't certain that I was completely convinced. So I made sure to give her a ring two months later, just to check.

"No, it still hasn't even come up for me, Brandon. I've got other stuff I need to handle, but the jealousy issue has definitely lost its hold over me."

What an extraordinary first experiment! Not only had Nancy successfully uncovered this that we all spend our lives seeking—the love and peace that is at the center of our being, that is our soul— but she had succeeded in getting to the very *core* of what was driving her jealousy game. She had been having jealous rages that felt completely out of control, but when she addressed the *real* issue, stored underneath it all—the fear of abandonment—and that was finally resolved, the jealousy was no longer even an issue for her!

"Interesting," I thought. "So it's possible to get to the core of an issue, to the very incidents that put it in place. Once the core issue is resolved, then the surface issue can finally free itself." I thought, "What if *everyone* was capable of this? What if we could all get to the *real* cause of our pain, and free ourselves BEFORE we create disease? What if we all could give ourselves our own wake-up calls, so that our bodies aren't required to do it all for us?"

Unlike Nancy, I had been given a huge wake-up call by my body—in the form of the tumor. And I wasn't given much time to uncover what my core issue was, what was stored there in the cells. Thank goodness I was guided to uncover those past issues, and finally release them, so that my body could go about the natural process of healing.

If only I'd given myself this wake-up call sooner. Perhaps then the tumor wouldn't have been created in the first place. Perhaps I might have freed myself before the degenerative cell pattern started.

14

And so I began to do my one-on-one therapy work with this unlayering principle in mind. I was determined to help people get underneath their surface issues, to the core of what was really "running their show" on an emotional level—and I knew it was essential for real transformation that it take place at the level of the soul.

So that the process could refine itself without professional pressures, I began by working with my closest friends and family members. I worked with any dear one who was open to self-discovery, and who sincerely longed to be free from an emotional issue that they felt hooked by—that seemed to be running on automatic pilot.

I knew that jealousy and abandonment were not the only emotional issues that drive us. We all have issues, and at one time or another it can feel like they control us. And yet, we've never known how to get to the real *core* of the issue—the underlying *cause* of the pain. And so we just approach it from the surface level, either ignoring it and pretending it doesn't exist, or trying to convince ourselves that if we say all the right things inside our heads about the issue, we might actually fix ourselves. Meanwhile, the *hidden cause* remains at our core, and we wonder why, no matter how hard we try, we somehow can't seem to let it go.

To a person, everyone I worked with dropped through the layers successfully, and then was dumbfounded that *old* wounds were the cause of their *current* pain. I was thrilled at the amazing results they achieved. We worked on everything from jealousy to resentment, fear, guilt, shame, loss, rage—you name it. Over the months I could see a clear pattern emerging, and so I decided to construct a very simple script that could be used to help people go down through the emotional layers. I then created another one to help people discover and resolve the emotional issues with the people at their campfire. It included a fireside chat, a complete forgiveness process, and yet another one for the "future integration"—so that they could see how things would be different in the future. This was followed by a letter from the future them to the present them.

As the script involved graphics, Nancy, who was a computer whiz, came over and put it all onto the computer for me, helping me get a clearer picture of the whole process. When it came off the printer, I handed it to Don, whom I knew was not only an expert in the field, but who was by nature quite critical and skeptical. After reading it through, he said, "This is impressive, Brandon. It's probably some of the deepest and most important work going on in the field of mind-body healing today. Do you mind if I start using it in some of my own private consultations?"

"No," I said, stunned and humbled by his response. I'd expected him to be quite critical and nitpicking. Instead, he seemed genuinely impressed.

He said, "You've put months of work into this, and it shows; not just in the wording, but in the whole syntax and content. It's not just remarkable, it's *usable*."

I was flabbergasted, and felt that perhaps some of the in-depth work I'd done over the last several months might have actually paid off. As we sat together on our living room sofa, and I flipped through the dozen pages of the first draft of "The Emotional Journey Process," I felt as if a piece of the puzzle had finally dropped into place. Resting in my hands was a "living" tool that could be used in a very practical way to help others go on their own spiritual and emotional journeys.

I quietly shared with Don what my vision with "The Emotional Journey Process" was; how deeply grateful I'd been for the tumor, and how that wake-up call had set me free on so many levels, not just physically. It had been a priceless gift that I felt somehow must be passed on to others, and I prayed that through it others might recognize the immense wisdom inherent in themselves, and be inspired to go on their own spiritual and physical journeys of discovery.

I told him how deeply moved I'd been over the last several months—how privileged I felt to be allowed to assist others in discovering their true selves, and how awed I was by everyone's success in setting themselves free. I'd been amazed by the soul's natural desire and willingness to help the body become free from the emotional issues that had been stored there for years. Everyone had been so open, so willing, so courageous, and the results reflected that greatness.

I'd once heard a spiritual teacher say, "If you take one step toward Grace, it will take a thousand steps toward you." It certainly seemed to be true in the case of healing. It feels as if the body wisdom is eager to assist us in letting go of these old issues: if we but make a small effort toward it, it does the rest.

I told Don that what I really longed for was to reach out to people who had *physical* challenges and blocks and disease, that I wanted to serve others in not only becoming free from emotional issues, but helping them go on a *physical* healing journey as well. From my own experience with the tumor, I'd seen how powerful it had been to uncover and discover the memories that were stored inside the cells, and get to the core of it all. And I intrinsically felt that this wasn't just a fluke experience unique to me. I knew that this possibility exists for all of us. And so silently, I put out a prayer that people who had physical challenges would be drawn to me so that we could begin working on that level, as well as the emotional level.

15

The next day, Don flew out to give one of his Robbins Research seminars in New York, and while he was there, a woman named Ruth called him and asked if he could help her. She had been diagnosed with a grapefruit-sized uterine tumor and, even though she was in her sixties, she didn't believe in the adage "you can't teach an old dog new tricks." She was very open to trying anything that might help her heal herself.

She had been told by doctors that her only option was surgery, and she would have to have her uterus taken out. She said, "You know, just because I've passed the childbearing age doesn't mean I want to have my womb removed. They seem so matter-of-fact about it, like I should think it was normal to have my insides cut out."

She'd heard through a friend that I'd been successful at healing myself from a tumor much bigger than hers, and she wondered if Don could give her any advice. She was due to go in for surgery in one month's time. Don warmly encouraged her, replying that it's never too late to learn, and that he definitely felt that it is possible to participate in your own healing. He suggested she give me a ring, to speak to me directly, and, after she had heard my story, he would help her in any way he could.

Only one day had gone by, and already my prayer was answering itself. People with physical challenges were being drawn to

"The Journey." Don forgot to call me to let me know he'd given her my number, so when she called it was a complete surprise. I was delighted to speak with her and said how strongly I admired her courage and openness, and I let her know that healing at a cellular level is definitely possible. I asked her what type of tumor it was, and she said that they thought it was fibroid.

"That's benign (noncancerous), isn't it?"

"Yeah," she said, in her crusty New York accent.

"So, is there any danger in postponing?"

"No. As a matter of fact, there really isn't. It's just . . . you know, doctors . . ."

I asked her if she would be willing to delay her next doctor's examination for at least six weeks.

"But I'm scheduled for surgery in one month."

"I know this is a big thing to ask, but could you *un*-schedule it, or postpone it, at the very least? It took me six weeks for the healing to complete itself, and I wouldn't want you to cut yourself short of time."

She sounded flustered and unsure. I'd been so clear-cut and forthright from our first sentence, and she was still grappling with the idea that her healing could take place that quickly. Then I filled her in on my own story, ending it with the suggestion that she see my husband for a one-on-one, where she would get a chance to undergo a physical process I'd developed out of my own healing experience. At the very least, she would emotionally free herself from what was stored inside the tumor, and learn the lessons it had to teach her.

She asked me if I'd done this process with anyone else who had a tumor, and I admitted that she would be the first other than myself, but assured her that all she had to lose were whatever limitations, old wounded patterns, and traumatic memories were stored inside her cells. At the very worst, she would only have wasted two hours of her time and postponed an operation that wasn't urgent. At the very best, she might succeed in freeing herself from the tumor.

We spoke for about forty-five minutes, and at the end she sounded grateful, but still somewhat skeptical. I couldn't blame her. I'm the same way. Unless I know something to be true and real for me, it can all sound like so many words.

She followed through, however—delayed her surgery by an extra month and made an appointment with Don. As it turned out, the doctors didn't give her the hassle she expected—maybe because they considered her case to be more routine than urgent.

Don called the following evening and asked, "Now, tell me again how it was you actually went into the tumor itself and uncovered the memories that were there?" I had recently completed work on a whole new version of the process I had originally undergone on the massage therapist's couch. Using language patterns friendly to the other-than-conscious mind, the Physical Journey guided people down a set of steps into their Source. While here, in their essence, they were asked, in their mind's eye, to step inside a magical space shuttle which was capable of taking them safely and gracefully to any part of the body— it was powered by their internal body wisdom, so there was nothing for them to think about or effort over. All they needed to do was to let *it* take them where *it* wanted to go.

In this way, we could be sure that *their own inner genius was allowed to be in control* of where the work would begin—it let their conscious minds off the hook in making that decision. The cell memories would be accessed in the place their inner intelligence, their body wisdom, chose, and the processing would take place there.

I briefed Don thoroughly in the new Physical Journey syntax, and made some specific suggestions about how to work with Ruth. Once he'd got clear, and sounded confident he could do the work with her, I said, "Funny, *you're* the one to do the first physical processing. Isn't it interesting that it would be with a woman who has a tumor in her uterus?"

"Yes, but she's in her sixties and doesn't have the background and understanding that you do, Brandon."

"Well, it's not the person, it's the *process* that works! Goodness knows we've certainly discovered that by now. Anyway, it won't be up to either you or Ruth; it'll be up to the infinite intelligence inside her body to do the actual healing. You guys will be just willing participants in the process. Call me when you've finished. Let me know how it goes."

Three days later, Don called. "Well, surprisingly, it went very well. She's got a lot of spunk for a lady in her sixties, and she really went for it. She says she'd like another session just to make sure."

"Sure, why don't you? It can't hurt; all she has to lose is some old emotional baggage." And so they had a second session.

We didn't hear from Ruth for three months. Robbins Research had sent us to Australia to give seminars, and so we missed the message she'd left on our machine. When we came back I was tickled to hear that husky New York accent coming over the answering machine.

"Well, I went to the doctors. They couldn't find the tumor; all that was left was a little fluid that they drained off with a needle . . . just thought you'd like to know. Guess we stumped them, huh?" She sounded droll, mildly playful, and somehow dryly unimpressed all at once.

16

While preparing for our trip to Australia, I continued to refine the Emotional Journey Process, taking into account all that I was continuing to learn when working with people. Each time I worked with someone the script got stronger, clearer, and more user-friendly. I decided to take the script with me to Australia, in case the need for Journeywork arose while I was there.

We had a wonderful time in Australia. The Aussies are always so welcoming and boisterous. It feels like such a newborn country, and there is a fresh enthusiasm and openness to their nature that I find particularly appealing.

While we were there, it occurred to me that these might be the very people who'd like to *learn* the Emotional Journey Process. It had been some twenty-one months since my tumor, and I'd worked with people only in one-to-one sessions. Although people had achieved hugely successful results, I still felt *I* was guiding them through the process, and they weren't actually *learning* the process itself. I was "giving them fish," but I wasn't "teaching them *how* to fish." I had often thought how much more empowering it would be if people could learn to do this process themselves. Then they wouldn't need to go to a specialized trainer or therapist to get the work done, but could continue their unlayering process on their own.

It is a Journey, after all! It's not like a sticking plaster, where we fix one issue and we're done. We all have many emotional issues to work on, and my real prayer is that we continue to let go of these limitations for as long as they come up for us. We should never stop transforming; just come ever more fully into the awareness of ourselves as this pristine diamond, always letting go of the limiting layers that seem to obscure us from our true selves.

I thought how wonderful it would be if I could *teach* people how to do the Emotional Journey Process together, and then they would have a set of skills to work with for any emotional issue that might come up in their lives. It's not as if I, personally, needed to be part of everyone's healing journey. It's preferable for people to peel back their own layers, discover the boundless silence of being that is their own self, resolve their own emotional issues, completely forgive and finish their own stories. Then it's up to nature to do what it knows how to do—heal the body *and* the being.

I thought, "Wouldn't it be wonderful if people could have a script to work with—one that they could share with their partners and loved ones. Rather than sit and watch television every night, maybe they might occasionally choose to do some transformative work with themselves, and begin to live as an expression of their true selves—as Freedom."

So I decided to put on a small evening workshop at the house of my close friends, Catherine and Peter. Their living room and drawing room areas could easily accommodate about sixteen people. I thought that would be a small but very manageable number to try out Journeywork with.

On the Sunday night of Don's final seminar, I put out a public invitation for people to come to this special first evening. I told my own story, and said I really only wanted to invite people who *sincerely* wished to be free from an issue they felt hooked by— some emotional pattern or physical challenge that, no matter how hard they'd tried, no matter how much therapy they'd done, no matter how many seminars they'd attended, it *still* kept coming up for them.

I didn't want to invite people who were just interested in learning yet another process. I only had sixteen spaces, and I felt those spaces were precious and should go to people who truly, deeply longed to be free from something that had been challenging them for years.

Half the room raised their hands, and so I had to reiterate my plea. "This is being done in service to freedom, and it's *not* a process for wimps or curiosity seekers. It's a process for those who really want to roll up their sleeves and look the tiger in the eye—face old emotional memories and patterns that may not be so comfortable to look at.

"I'm asking that only those prepared to do deep work, who feel ready to finally finish their stories, come to the back of the room to see me."

The places were filled as quickly as my pen could write. As I looked at a sea of disappointed faces, I felt terrible to have to turn everyone else away. I'd never realized how deeply we all long to know our true selves. And how much we long to let go of the shackles that emotionally bind us and keep us from experiencing the boundless joy at the core of our being.

I had already done the Journey process with a couple of dear friends in Australia, so I trained them to be helpers in order that the people doing Journeywork for the first time would feel very supported. Don was there alongside me, offering his immense expertise at that first Journey workshop. There were only eight couples working, and four of us helping, which seemed very manageable—one trained helper for every two couples working. There would be one of us on hand any time someone needed assistance, or if anyone had a question. I wanted everyone to know that it was a safe and nurturing environment, and that they were highly supported.

I was surprised that all sixteen people were either early, or arrived right on time. As everyone gathered together, I could feel an eagerness building, but also a lot of nervousness. I asked everyone to take a few minutes to let our energies settle, to let ourselves become "present." We closed our eyes and sat quietly together for silent meditation.

I found myself resting in the powerful peace that had become the familiar undercurrent of my life. The entire room fell silent in the profound presence of stillness. You could hear a pin drop. Not a muscle stirred, and yet there was an alertness, a scintillation to the energy in the room.

I felt as if my own awareness filled not only the room, but extended boundlessly beyond, encompassing everything and *in* everything. My mind became utterly still, completely thought free, and it seemed as if we were all bathing, soaking in this presence of love. We were steeping in Source.

After a few minutes we opened our eyes, and as I got ready to speak, it occurred to me that this stillness is contagious. If there is just one person hanging out in thought-free awareness, everyone "catches" it. I have since read a beautiful quotation by W. B. Yeats which expresses this perfectly:

> We can make our mind so like still water that beings gather about us to see their own images, and so for a moment live a clearer, perhaps even fiercer, life because of our quiet.

Over the years, I'd heard a Sanskrit word that was often used to describe this phenomenon. It's called *Satsang; Sat* means "truth," and *sang* means "in the company of." So *Satsang* means "in the company of truth," or in the presence of, or in the community of truth. Here we were resting in peace, in stillness, in the company of truth itself. *Satsang*.

After meditation, I told everyone of my healing journey, and even while the story was unfolding, we were still bathing in that peace, in *Satsang*. I made sure I included my experience of peeling back the layers and finding that underneath all the emotional layers was a black void of nothingness, and how, when I'd fallen through that "gateway," I had come into the extraordinary presence of love that I realized is my own soul. I shared with them the awe I felt in experiencing my own inner wisdom, and how I felt it was the infinite intelligence inside that was responsible for all the healing, and that I was only a humble participant in the process.

I shared that I felt it was possible for all beings to come to know their true selves, and in the realization of that, to then tap into the inner wisdom that springs naturally from their Source. I emphasized that Journeywork was not a mind-over-matter process, but rather a journey of discovery into the soul.

I told them I believed that real healing starts at the soul level— at the level of essential awareness—and reflects back through the emotional level to the physical level. So in order to get to the *core* of an emotional issue, we have to first get to the *core* of who we *really* are. Then, once we are in touch with our own essence, *that* wisdom can guide us to uncover what emotional memories are stored in the body. It's only then that we can get to the bottom of it all, and set ourselves free. As I spoke, I looked deeply into the eyes of the people listening, and was encouraged to see that some part of them seemed to recognize and understand what I was talking about.

I asked one of my friends, Ian, if he would be willing to do a live demonstration of the Journey process, and he warmly consented. He had an issue of frustration that had been bugging him, so we decided to use that. Although we were in Australia, Ian is English, and a little reserved. So, I was very grateful that he was emotionally open and authentic going down through the levels.

As he went down through the layers, it felt as if everyone in the room was going down through the levels with him. At one point he got to a layer of helplessness and, when he started to cry, I noticed that there were tears in a number of people's eyes. He had some slight resistance as he went into the black hole, which he called nothingness, and then his face began to beam with a radiant joy as he came into the presence of peace within.

He ended up with an early childhood memory, of when he was

in the crib. He felt he'd been abandoned, and felt very frustrated and powerless that he couldn't communicate his need for help. Finally, at his campfire, he was able to express to his parents how he really felt at the time, and forgiveness came quite easily to him. When we'd finally finished the whole process, he looked quietly aglow and openly childlike.

I looked around the room, and tears were coming to several people's eyes. They felt so moved, so touched to see such profound transformation in such a brief period of time. In the room was a palpable tenderness and compassion combined with a willing openness that made it the perfect moment to suggest that people take out their scripts, pair up, and begin their own processes.

As I walked about the two rooms, I was deeply moved by the profundity of people's processes, and how much they let go of. There was one woman, though, who seemed to be having a difficult time going down through the layers—every time she got near the blackness she would avoid it and go right back up to where she started.

I noted that and thought, "Hmm, don't we all do this? Just when we are about ready to break through, something inside stops us, we get stuck and instead we run our old habits over and over again. We have a fear of the unknown, and will avoid it at any cost, even if it means never becoming free from our old stories of pain and suffering."

This woman had been diagnosed with chronic depression, and was so debilitated by it that she was unable to work and had been living on disability income for six years. She said to me when she arrived that night that this might be her last hope. She'd tried everything, from therapy to drugs to seminars, and nothing had worked for her. Even getting up in the morning was a struggle. As it was, she had dragged herself to this evening's workshop.

In her voice was the sound of failure, as if she had predetermined that she would fail this time, as she had done at every other attempt over the last six years. When I went over to her, she had already "cycled" three times—she just couldn't face the black hole. When I looked at what her partner had written down as her emotional layers, I thought, "Hmm, this is her whole pattern of depression perfectly laid out in black and white. It's classic. Of course she doesn't know how to drop through the black hole—it is the thing she fears most."

I recalled my own first experience of the black void, and remembered how I feared that I was on the brink of annihilation and how terrified I had been. I felt a deep compassion for her, yet a firm *knowing* that in order for her to finally break free from her old pattern she would *have* to face the blackness and fall through.

In a gentle but firm voice I said, "Do you recognize this old pattern? You go from depression to hopelessness, to helplessness, to desolation, to despair, to anxiety, to fear, and then you come to this black nothingness and get *stuck*, and feel angry and frustrated. Then what do you do? You get depressed at the frustration—then you go right back up to the top and run this whole pattern again. Is this something you do a lot in your life?"

"Oh, yes. It's an old friend of mine. I know it well. It's all I ever do, in fact. When I get to the anxiety and fear I give up. Then I get so frustrated I get depressed all over."

I asked if she finally wanted to be free. She said feistily, "Of course I do. I'm sick of this."

"Well, you're going to have to face that blackness and surrender into it, and just relax and finally drop through it."

"But I don't know what will happen to me if I do."

"I know," I said. "But if you want to be free, you'll just have to TRUST."

So, I guided her down through the layers, making sure she didn't linger too long at any level, as she had a tendency to wallow a bit, and I didn't want that to be a distraction to her. The Journey is not about expressing and wallowing in your pain at every level; it's about feeling the emotion long enough to taste it and drop through to the next level until you finally get down through all the layers to your Source.

When she got to the black hole, she announced in an "I told you so" voice, "I'm stuck!"

"So what if you were to relax and smile and just fall right into the blackness? What would that be like?"

"I don't know what that would be like!"

"But I wonder what it would be like if you did."

A brief look of confusion and questioning crossed her face, then she began shaking, "I'm falling! I'm falling!"

"Keep falling," I said. And suddenly she burst into tears, sobbing and sobbing, tears streaming. "I'm love . . . I'm God . . . it's God . . . it's . . . I don't know what it is. . . . I'm Free . . . I'm Freedom . . . I'm beautiful . . . it's beautiful . . ." She wept in relief, and beamed with awe.

I knew then that the rest of the process would be a piece of cake for her. She'd finally come to know what was underneath all that anxiety and fear, and she'd realized that there genuinely was nothing to fear. I handed the script back to her partner, and they finished the process successfully.

As the evening continued a couple of other people in the room felt a little reticent, and would raise their hands to ask questions, but all they really needed was a bit of reassurance from someone who'd actually been through the process.

Source really is contagious, and I had been aware for some time that when I was deeply immersed in Stillness, in Silence, whomever I was working with found their way into that awareness with greater ease and alacrity. To work with someone, you can't just do the process, you have to BE it, live it. Then it is easy for people to "catch it" from you.

I've carried this principle directly into my seminars. I give more and more advanced training to the assistants. When we work with people we really can assist them through a process fully. We've all been through it a number of times; we've seen the kinds of challenges that might come up, and we've developed skills in handling these challenges, and we're of much greater service to the people being processed.

When the evening workshop was over, it was well after midnight, yet people kept hanging about. No one wanted to leave. We all were basking in the healing afterglow of being in the pure presence of Love itself.

Three months later I received a letter postmarked from Australia. "Odd," I thought, "I didn't give anyone my address that night. This person must have gone through a lot of hassle trying to get my home address." When I opened it, I recognized the name at the bottom to be the lady who had been diagnosed with the chronic depression. My heart began to pound as I thought, "Oh no, did something happen?" until I read her simple but moving words.

She said that on the night of the Journey workshop, she uncovered an overwhelming anxiety *beneath* the blanket of depression. Once she faced and resolved the anxiety issue, the depression finished completely—she hadn't experienced a moment of depression since. She said that in the past it would have taken a gargantuan effort just to get out of bed in the morning, whereas now, not only was she naturally rising early, she was "simply and effectively going about her day." She was delighted to finally be back at work after six years of chronic illness.

Her letter now rests among thousands like it, in a huge file that I keep as a testament to the enormous courage and immense wisdom inherent in the human soul. Each time I receive a letter I am newly inspired and deeply moved—awed by the fearlessness, strength, and wisdom within us all, and it feels as if I'm hearing again for the first time what amazing Grace exists inside our own hearts. These letters still bring tears to my eyes—the greatness within never ceases to fill me with awe.

Out of that simple, intense first night, the Journey workshop expanded and refined itself. It has since grown into a full, rich and profoundly intensive two-day program where people leave in recognition of who they really are—having drunk deeply from this well of peace that is at the core of our being.

On day one we undergo the Emotional Journey. We learn and

experience the unlayering process and come into the core of our soul. Then our inner wisdom guides us to discover and resolve old emotional issues. We learn the campfire process and the future integration.

On the second day we all undergo the Physical Journey, a wondrous journey of discovery inside the body to uncover any blockages or rigid places or diseased areas that might exist. Then we discover the actual memories stored inside the cells, and go through the process of resolving them and doing the forgiveness work necessary to finish the story and set ourselves free.

So, would *you* like to have your own direct experience of the Emotional Journey process? You can stop reading now, or continue and do the process later. The script I use in the seminars is at the back of this book in the "Tools" section. You'll need to set aside a couple of hours of private time with a friend you trust, preferably one who has already read this book and is open and willing to work with you.

17

So, now that you've learned about or experienced the Emotional Journey process, it's time to learn more about the Physical Journey.

There is one man whose Physical Journey process was particularly moving. Jim was a humble baker, aged sixty-seven, who owned a small bakery in the north of England. His niece had come to one of my introductory seminars and had suggested to him that he might like to speak with me privately about his health condition. When she called to ask if I would see him, she warned me—"Jim is not familiar with all this mind-body healing stuff, and he can be very skeptical and independent minded. He's a Yorkshireman and has quite a fiery temper. I don't want you to feel intimidated by him."

I chuckled and said I would be happy to meet him. I explained that often, when people don't know about the work, they are actually a lot easier to work with.

"I don't know," she hesitated. "He can be pretty strong-willed."

"Strong wills are healthy things to have. Sounds like I'm going to like him!"

Jim traveled all the way down to London by train, not knowing anything about me, not even my story—just trusting the advice of his favorite niece. When I opened the door to welcome Jim, I looked into fierce blazing eyes and fiery red cheeks. Jim was just as Suzy had described him. It was clear he was a no-nonsense man, who definitely had a mind of his own.

With a determined stride he walked directly into my sitting room, and sat down before I even had a chance to offer him a seat. I liked him instantly. There was a twinkle in his eye, and behind his fierceness, I detected an inner radiance, a glow.

When we sat down for tea, he wasted no time in getting to the point. In his forthright Yorkshire manner he said, "I don't know what it is you do, but my niece seems to think you might be able to help me." I readied myself to give him a condensed version of my own story, and began with, "Well, actually . . ." But before I could get the words out, he abruptly interrupted with, "No, no! I want to tell you *my* story . . ." Then, with a twinkle in his eye, he said, "I showed them . . . I showed them all."

My interest was piqued. I asked what he meant, and it gave him the exact opening he was looking for, as, with great gusto, he launched headlong into his story.

"Two years ago I went to see my family doctor. He sat me down as if to have a heart-to-heart chat with me, looked me straight in the eyes, put on a grave voice, and said they'd found an egg-size cancerous tumor in my lung. It was so far advanced that I had less than three months to live. He said there was nothing they could do for me, and that I needed to get my affairs in order.

"Can you imagine that?" Jim bellowed, obviously outraged. "A doctor telling me I have only three months to live! What a load of crap! I'm not ready to kick the bucket yet—it's not my time to die! I may have lung cancer, but that doesn't mean I'm willing to pack it in and give up. What a load of rubbish—bloody hell!"

"So, what happened," I asked, intrigued by this time. I was absolutely enthralled by his garrulous manner.

"Well . . . I found another doctor."

"What did he say?" I asked.

"He said I had only *two* months left to live!"

"So, what did you do?"

"What else could I do? I sacked him. Then I found a third doctor, and I sacked him too."

"Then what happened?"

"Well . . . finally I found a doctor who made some sense. She had a history of successful cases, and had actually succeeded in helping seven people go into remission from the very same type of cancer I had. I figured she would be worth listening to, because at least she knew that it was possible to survive and heal. She was the first doctor I came to who wasn't convinced that I had to die."

As I watched this sixty-seven-year-old baker, I felt such a sense of admiration. He had such a feisty fighting spirit and a crusty, wry sense of humor. He had no background in the field of health, and yet he knew that you don't have to take your first prognosis. I thought how wonderful it would be if we all had this strong will to live. What an example he is to all of us.

I'd read in several books about the psychology of the patients who survive cancer. One of the most important qualities that researchers determined was a causal factor in survival was this strong will to live. Often the most difficult patients, who are most cantankerous and trying for the doctors and demanding of the nurses, are the very ones that beat the odds. Here was such a man.

"So, what happened, Jim? You obviously didn't kick the bucket!" He looked like a picture of health, and I told him just that. He went on to describe the various treatments he had undergone: chemotherapy, radiation, etc. There was a genuine sense of pride in his voice when he finished his story with "I showed them all. Three months ago I had an MRI scan (soft tissue X-ray) and the diagnosis was good. The tumor has gone into remission—it didn't metastasize as they expected—it hasn't spread."

His face looked all aglow, and he chuckled as he added, "A couple of months ago I ran into that first doctor. Was he in for a shock when he saw me! He turned completely pale, as if he'd seen a ghost. He was absolutely convinced I'd died twenty months ago! And I don't plan on stopping now—I'm going to *keep* on going!" From the spirit of the man who sat before me, I knew he would. He stubbornly and triumphantly punctuated the end of his story with, "My time is not up yet!"

I said, "This is an incredible story, Jim. You should go out there and share it with people. Let them know it's possible to participate in their own healing journey, that you don't have to take the first prognosis you get as gospel, and that we all have the freedom to choose which healing path we wish to take. You should go out there and talk to other patients with your type of cancer. Let them see the possibility right before their own eyes. You are a wonderful example to us all."

"Oh, I know that. I'm already doing that in my own way," he shrugged, a little embarrassed.

"So why are you here?" I asked. "I feel like you are a teacher for me. You are such a shining example of what's possible."

All of a sudden, his gregarious, almost boisterous manner became very quiet and vulnerably tender. His voice became almost inaudible, and his face became childlike and open. I had to lean forward to hear the words that explained his visit.

"I want to know why . . . I want to know why *this* is here," he whispered, tapping his chest. "I know I'm meant to learn something from all of this. This didn't happen just so I could prove some doctors wrong. I know it happened for a reason. I just want to know why," he said, tenderly, almost plaintively. "I don't want it showing up in some other part of my body just because I didn't learn what it had to teach me."

I was arrested by his words. Tears came to my eyes to be in the presence of so much strength and courage, and such obvious humility all at once. This man was showing me that he was willing to admit he didn't have all the answers, and he hoped that maybe I could point him toward discovering what it was the tumor had to teach him. I felt so touched by his tender exposure I couldn't speak for a moment or two.

Then, very simply, I replied, "Well, that's my speciality. I help people uncover what it is that these diseases have to teach us. It's my prayer that if we really *learn* the lessons, we won't have to repeat them. My belief is that the reason so many people have the experience of having a cancerous tumor surgically removed, and then, three years later, another one shows up somewhere else, is because they didn't learn the lessons, and get the understanding the soul wanted to give them the first time around. So then the soul says 'Hey, you didn't listen to my first wake-up call—let me try again. Maybe you'll listen this time.' And so another tumor pops up."

Jim agreed. He said, "Oh, I'm sure I'm meant to learn something. I just don't know what."

And so I told him a very brief version of my own story, ending it with the statement that I'd be happy to help him uncover the old memories stored inside that tumor, so he could learn what it was the tumor had to teach him. He looked deeply into my eyes, as if searching my soul, and then said quietly, "I still don't know what it is you do, but I trust you and I'm willing to try anything."

And so we began the Physical Journey process. Here was a man who knew nothing about mind-body anything, who just somehow knew that there was something deeper to understand. Once again I thought to myself how thirsty we all are to learn our lessons and become free. What a divine thirst that is.

For such a strong, stalwart man he turned out to be very open and very real in his process. He was almost childlike in his openness. When he arrived inside his lung, before I could ask him what was there in the tumor, a *very vivid* memory flashed before him.

He was sixteen years old, in wartime England. His father had already deserted the family, and left him to care for his mother. German bombs were being dropped all over the country. He was at school when a bomb landed in his section of town. Something inside him panicked. Fighting the schoolmasters, he broke free, ran out of his school, and ran home to find his mother. Searching, searching . . . she was not there.

Finally, he ran through the side lanes into the high street. There he found her. She lay perfectly stretched out, young and beautiful, as if just lying down for a nap. Her clothes looked perfect, as if they'd been "ironed onto her." He ran over to her, and tried to shake her awake. He kept shaking her and shaking her, until finally the police came and pulled them apart.

"She's dead, son."

Then the tears and the rage came. A rage he could never express—a rage against God. How could he ever forgive God for taking his mother before her time? She was so young, so beautiful, so full of life. How could God do this? What kind of God does this?

More rage came—rage against the enemy. How could he ever forgive those evil Nazis? She didn't have a gun. She wasn't even in the war. How could they kill an innocent woman? How could he find compassion for a people so evil? All the unexpressed, unre-solvable *rage* just came pouring out. So, young Jim, not knowing what to do with all the pain, stuffed it right there beside his heart—in his left lung.

I suggested something I'd never done before. I asked Jim to set up a campfire right there inside his lung, and to invite all the people in his memory, *including God,* for a fireside chat. I sat silently as Jim expressed fifty years of unspoken rage against God, finally speaking his piece, getting it off his chest and out of his cells.

I asked him what he thought God might reply, and it seemed as if an inner wisdom arose from somewhere deep inside of him. It explained that no one can be taken before their time. There were other plans for his mom, and he should know that she is at peace and exactly where she needs to be. Then when it was time for him to forgive God, it seemed as if his heart broke wide open, and a profound forgiveness poured from him, a forgiveness so huge it took my breath away. His humility and love brought me to my knees.

Then he spoke to the Nazis. He expressed such a heart-rending rage that I didn't know if my own heart could bear it. And, once again, when he asked the inner wisdom why, the enemy replied that they were just acting under orders, and that they were just as scared as he. Guns were being pointed at their heads, and their mothers were dying as well.

Compassion poured from Jim as he wept in complete understanding of their plight. His voice broke as he forgave the enemy with all his heart. Then he actually asked for their forgiveness for having so wrongly judged them for all these years.

I could see that he was finally complete. It was over. Fifty years of unresolved rage had finished. He looked as if a cement mask had broken wide open, revealing the real him underneath, and he shone with a quiet radiance.

When his process was over, I sat quietly with this extraordinary man. A childlike innocence and peace seemed to radiate from him. Quietly, I said, "I was right. You came here as *my* teacher." His face was flushed and his eyes sparkled like diamonds, and a quiet inner sweetness poured from him. There was not much more to say.

Before he got up to leave, I thanked him for coming, and said, "I know you're getting another MRI scan in two weeks' time. I'd like to ask you to stay open to the possibility that they might not find anything there."

"Oh, no, no," he said, quite surprised that I would suggest such a thing. "It can't happen. You see, my tumor's not like yours, it's a different type. There is no recorded history of *anyone* who has had this kind of tumor disappear. With lung cancer the best you can hope for is that it goes into remission—that it doesn't spread, and it's already done that. I didn't come to you to *heal* the tumor. I just came to you to find out why it was there, and to learn what it had to teach me."

I said softly, "Well, why not just stay open to the possibility— maybe you'll be the first. You never know. Just keep on being the shining example you already are. Go out and spread the word that healing at a cellular level is possible. It was such an honor to work with you." As he left, I thought what an immense blessing it is to be allowed to do this work. I have to be the luckiest person alive. Truly, for me, it doesn't feel so much like work, it feels like a privilege.

Three weeks went by, and no news from Jim. I was a little disappointed not to hear from him. Then I got a phone call from his niece, Suzy. All ebullient and enthusiastic, she said, "My aunt is wondering what you did to my uncle. Jim's become a pussycat! He's no longer raging about the place—barking at the help when they spill the flour, or blowing his stack when the loaves don't come out right. He's no longer yelling at the traffic, or angry at the news. He's become so much sweeter and kinder. My aunt asked me to thank you. She feels like she's finally got the man that she knew was there when she first married him forty-five years ago."

I laughed and said I was delighted to hear the news, and shared briefly with her what a privilege it was to have worked with her uncle. I kept waiting for her to mention the MRI scan. It was clear the conversation was coming to an end, and she still hadn't mentioned it. Finally, as we were getting ready to say our goodbyes, I found the nerve to ask the question, "So, what happened with Jim's MRI scan?"

"Oh, yeah. They didn't find anything. All that was left was a hairline scar," she replied.

"That's amazing! What are the doctors saying about it?"

"It's like a circus at the hospital. They're all going nuts trying to figure it out. Half the medical team is certain that they must have misdiagnosed him in the first place, and the other half is trying to attribute it to a drug he was given two years ago. They're treating Jim like a 'lab rat,' giving him every test on the planet. He's the first recorded case where a cancerous lung tumor actually disappeared."

"How's Jim taking it?" I asked.

"You know Jim . . . He takes it all with a pinch of salt and a big dose of humor."

A week later, I received a joyous and moving letter from Suzy detailing his remarkable progress. After reading this letter, I thought, "You know, we all go on our own spiritual and healing journeys, each in a different way. This man chose radiation and chemotherapy, and fortunately he also got the lessons his soul wanted him to learn. He needed to become free from fifty years of rage. What a lesson to learn."

We all think, "It's the traffic that makes me angry," or "It's the news that pisses me off," or "If only so-and-so would get it right, I wouldn't have to blow up at him." We think what causes our anger is something outside of us, when in truth, the anger is already stored inside. Those outer circumstances just push our button, and activate the emotion that was there all along. The anger button is not the only button we have. A whole host of buried emotions are stored inside us, and our outer circumstances are merely triggers that activate what is already stored inside.

Sometimes I think diseases can turn out to be our greatest gifts. For Jim, it was the gift of letting go of fifty years of rage, which finally gave him back his real Self. The doctors still can't explain the miracle of his tumor's disappearance. I heard from an independent source that Jim's case has now been published in a British medical journal, and the tumor's disappearance has been attributed to the drug he took two years before doing the Physical Journey process.

18

One of my favorite aspects of Journeywork is the profound healing and forgiveness that takes place *within* families, after completing their Journey processes.

Journeywork is *not* about uncovering memories so that we can
use them to justify our current behavior, or to use as a weapon to
blame those we love. The Journey is about *resolving* our issues,
healing the pain, *completing* the stories and *forgiving* those we love,
so that we can get on with our lives healthily—free from the
emotional baggage of the past.

There is one woman whose courageous story epitomizes the
depth of forgiveness possible, and the powerful effect it can have
on healing an entire family. Rachel was a warmhearted, thirty-
two-year-old mother whose story is not unlike that of many people who have been diagnosed with chronic depression.

Adopted at age two-and-a-half, she had been repeatedly sexu-
ally and physically abused by her adoptive family and their friends
throughout early childhood. Like most children in her circumstances, she didn't have the emotional coping skills to deal with
the unbearable trauma and distress it caused. Depression became
a blanket to numb her to the pain.

By the age of eleven she was in her first therapist's chair. At
sixteen her internal suffering was still unresolved and so unbearable that she made the first of several attempts to take her own

life. She had been in and out of doctors' and psychiatrists' offices and hospital psychiatric wards, with stress, breakdowns and depressive bouts, ever since. She had taken every imaginable sedative and antidepressant drug, but no amount of therapy or medication freed her from the despair.

Her three beautiful children were taken from her and put into foster care, as she was diagnosed as emotionally unfit to be a mother. Even with heavy doses of sleeping pills, she was managing only two hours of sleep per night. She felt she was spiraling down into a hopelessness from which there would be no return.

She wrote me a heartrending letter telling me of her amazing return to health since her first Journey process. She said she had not seen a great improvement for a few days. Then one night she decided she did not need the temazepam to get to sleep. She slept solidly for eight hours. "It was absolutely wonderful. No nightmares, nothing. I could have run around shouting for joy."

She started looking at herself differently. She actually started to smile, something she hadn't done for over two years. She went and saw her mother, and had a long chat with her. "After so many years it was wonderful to be able to hug her and tell her that I loved her, and that I really did forgive her for what she had done to me."

She stopped taking the Prozac and hasn't touched it since, saying her life feels whole again. She ended with the news that she had finally got her children back. They all attended a Journey children's retreat together, and it was so moving to see them reunited, playing so naturally together in such a loving environment.

Sean, her son, ended up being one of the "stars" of the kids' program, admired by both children and adults alike. He and his brother underwent much of the same kind of powerful and profound healing process work that Rachel had, and they also let go of years of emotional pain.

Together, they are a joyous example of how even the most hopeless-seeming family circumstances can be healed.

19

For me, one of the most rewarding aspects of Journeywork is when whole families go through the healing process. In this way healing on all levels can take place as the family grows together. It doesn't seem to matter how old or how young someone is—the soul longs to set us free.

Children can be such examples of openness and willingness to heal. They put up very few barriers or resistances, and so transformation comes very easily for them. I love working with them. They are such teachers. At the children's workshop, the Junior Journey, there is one trainer-supervisor for every two to three children. But I think it's often the children who teach the grownups how *easy* it is to let go and forgive the pain of the past. Unlike many resistant adults, they don't make it into such a "big deal."

I've worked with children who, after they've completed Journeywork, go skipping down the hall, singing, running out to the garden, joyfully playing, embracing life without looking back for even one moment to linger or wallow in past pain.

So often, young children hang out in Source spontaneously, so for them the Journey process comes naturally—it's barely work at all. They have a way of making it fun and playful. They are quick to forgive, and they don't have their identities and egos tied up in having to be consistent with their old limiting patterns and habits. They are thrilled to be free, and they trust they'll be healed easily.

Usually, their favorite process is the Physical Journey. In it they go into the imaginary magical space shuttle which carries them safely into whatever part of the body needs healing. It can go anywhere—into organs, veins, arteries, blood, tissues, bones, and so on—anywhere inside the body. Once they have arrived they take out big flashlights and look around. They love this part and can be quite graphic in their descriptions of the internal organs. I'm amazed at how often small children will describe a certain organ precisely, almost to a tee. It's particularly extraordinary when they have never studied anatomy.

They take with them a hero or a guardian angel who helps to uncover the memories stored in the cells. Once they've discovered a memory, they put the whole scene up onto a movie screen, and let it play from beginning to end. Then they invite the people in the memory to step down off the screen, come over to a campfire, and receive balloons full of empowering, resourceful states that would have helped them at the time the memory took place.

So, the younger child that went through the traumatic memory is given a whole balloon bouquet of resourceful states—like courage, strength, the ability to communicate and express their true feelings, honesty, truth, creativity, lightheartedness, a sense of humor, confidence, self-worth, understanding, compassion, joy, love, the ability to ask for help from the right people, and a "crystal dome" that lets other people's hurtful behavior roll off them, and so on.

Then, armed with this huge balloon bouquet of internal resources, the child steps back onto the movie screen and plays the scene *the way it would have happened* if they'd had access to these helpful states at the time. The child sees how, in summoning forward their best qualities, the scene plays itself out with much greater ease. This little process is actually quite powerful, as the child learns that he or she has strong resources already inside to draw on in similar circumstances in the future.

Once the *new* scene has been played out and they've experienced the new, more resourceful states, all the people in the memory are invited to step down off the screen and come over to the campfire for a fireside chat. The child finally gets a chance to express what was truly felt at the time. They get it off their chest and out of their cells. And, like the adults, they then go through the forgiveness work, but instead of using the word forgiveness, we call it the "I'm sorry, it's okay" process. Even very young children seem to understand its meaning and feel very little resistance to genuinely forgiving.

After the whole process is complete they take out their imaginary flashlights and look around the organ. It's extraordinary how quickly they see the cells beginning to change and how colorful they are in their descriptions.

I can remember one child who had a sore throat before he began his Physical Journey. When he took his space shuttle into his throat and took out his flashlight, it looked all rough and sandy. In his process he uncovered a memory where he was on holiday in Spain with his parents. He'd got lost and thought they'd forgotten him. He didn't know how to ask for help, and was feeling quite panicked. Eventually his parents showed up, but he never told them how frightened he was. During his campfire chat, it was very freeing for him to finally express to his parents how upsetting it had all been. He really got it all off his chest.

While at the campfire, his parents apologized. He came to realize that in fact they'd never *actually* left him; they'd just gone off for a short period of time. The "I'm sorry, it's okay" process was sweet, and very complete. At the end of the forgiveness process, when he checked around with his big flashlight, he found his throat no longer looked rough and sandy, but pink and smooth. And when his Physical Journey was over, the soreness in his throat had completely disappeared.

Isn't it interesting that once he finally communicated his true feelings by *speaking* them out loud, his throat was no longer sore? Another young child at the children's workshop hadn't spoken a single word since the death of one of his parents, several months earlier. As he couldn't speak during his Physical Journey process,

Freya, the advanced trainer heading the children's program, got him to signal to her what was taking place. He would indicate with his hands where he was in the body, and signal yes or no to the questions she asked. Freya's expertise and creativity combined with the Physical Journey script, which reads almost like a guided fairy tale, enabled them to successfully complete the process.

Amazingly, at the end of his session he spoke his first words in several months. He explained to Freya that because of the suddenness of his father's death he'd not been able to say goodbye to him. While at the campfire together, he and his father shared what they hadn't been able to say at the time of the death, and the young boy finally "completed" with his dad. His father assured him that he was always there for him, was always watching over him, and that his love would always be planted in his son's heart. Ever since his process he's been speaking fluently, and has been able to get on with his life more healthfully.

Another boy came quite reluctantly to the kids' workshop. His mother was one of our assistants, and he felt she had "dragged" him along. He had had problems with dyslexia and wasn't doing well at school, and his mother Jenny shared with us that the teachers had called her to let her know that Nathan would most likely *not* pass his exams. She felt crushed and brought him to the workshop to see if it could possibly help him in some way.

At first he was resistant, but soon became a positive model for the younger children. He became a mentor—older brother figure for one of the five-year-old girls, and they developed a special friendship, which brought out his self-confidence.

The next week in school, much to the amazement of his teachers, he ended up passing his exams with flying colors. His mother was even more surprised that the following weekend his confidence and skill level in his tennis game increased dramatically. Most surprising of all, even though he had been quite short for his age, he had a sudden growth spurt. Jenny remarked that the change in Nathan was so dramatic that she couldn't believe how self-assured he seemed.

Brett, the father of one of the Junior Journey graduates, wrote this beautiful letter about his son:

> . . . I would like to give you some feedback about my son Richard. I brought him to the November children's workshop. The issue I hoped would surface was his lack of self-confidence.
>
> Last Wednesday, Mary and I attended his first Parents' Evening at his new school. Without exception, the teachers commented, without prompting, that they had noticed a huge improvement in his self-confidence. This, in turn, was having a positive effect on his work.
>
> When we came home and mentioned this to Richard, his immediate reaction was, "It was all because of Brandon's workshop."

The stories from the children's workshops are as myriad and miraculous as children are. The children sing inspiring songs with lyrics about their own freedom, love, and forgiveness, and they share their success stories from their process work.

I am always moved by their artwork. They paint pictures before their process work and they paint pictures after it. The contrast is mind-blowing. Usually the "before" pictures are very sad and bleak-looking, and are painted in blacks, reds, and dark blues. The little cartoon faces often have tears coming down their cheeks. The "after" pictures usually are done in bright sunny colors—yellow, pink and orange. Usually, they have big suns and colorful flowers. Everyone in the pictures wears big bright smiles. It's such a profound contrast!

During the workshop the children uncover what inner qualities *they* have that are like the qualities of a hero, and they get a chance to practice these qualities with the other children. They receive actual balloons with resourceful qualities written on them, like courage, love, kindness, honesty, goodness, fun, forgiveness, and then they undergo several interactive team-building processes where they get a chance to demonstrate these heroic qualities.

I love seeing these "young brave heroes" going out into the world thinking it's actually "cool" to be kind or "hip" to be caring or "happening" to be generous. My prayer for children is that they live as a true expression of their own essence—so that they don't have to create the limiting emotional baggage that leads to so much of the physical blockages and disease patterns common to adults.

My belief is that if you live as a true expression of your Self, your soul, you don't have to co-create disease. With these children, I really feel that they get a healthy head start and I pray that they take the work and continue to use it. The truth is, we are all children inside. Wouldn't it be wonderful if we could follow their example and trust that letting go can be easy and fun?

If your heart feels called to work with your child, there are special instructions for working with children at the back of this book.

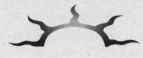

20

In various cities around the world, graduates have formed support groups that meet once a month. These meetings have been very popular and are a supportive way to continue letting go of the emotional veils that seem to obscure our "diamonds." It is great to work with others who have the same skills and who are willing to see us for who we *really* are.

Have you ever had the experience of feeling that you've grown as a person, then gone back to visit relatives who treat you like the person you *used* to be? Even though you feel like you've progressed, they seem to hold on to their outdated image of you. No matter how hard you try to communicate from your new perspective, they continue to see you in the old way.

At the grad meetings, I find it so liberating that we are all willing to greet each other freshly, with new eyes. We know everyone is evolving, and we refuse to hold on to past impressions. We continually ask the question, "Who's showing up, right now?" And I often ask graduates, "What would you rather do—sit around and watch television, or sit together and spend a couple of hours setting yourself free emotionally?" It really can be that easy.

At one grad support meeting I attended in Manchester, England, Anita, a lady in her fifties, piped up to share her story. She said that she had attended the Journey weekend workshop three weeks earlier and truthfully didn't expect a physical result. She'd had chronic acute knee pain for years, and it had become so bad it was hard for her to push the clutch down, or even walk to her car. She said, "I thought, Brandon may be able to heal herself, but not me. All I want is the emotional freedom." But she persevered nonetheless and did two Physical Journeys.

With a huge smile on her face she said, "Honestly, I didn't expect a result and I didn't actually notice any difference after I did the process. But just yesterday it dawned on me—I'm *squatting* in my garden weeding. I couldn't even have kneeled before, let alone squatted. I hadn't realized my knee had actually healed—it seemed so natural to be squatting again, I didn't even think about it."

Only three weeks had gone by since her process. Later she sent me the following letter:

Dear Brandon,

In 1991, I was walking in deep snow in Austria, when I injured my left knee, making walking difficult and painful. Even after physiotherapy it never fully recovered, and each year I have been forced to give up yet another activity that I loved—first circle dancing, then hill walking.

This year the deterioration was so much worse that in desperation I went to the doctor. She merely stated that I had arthritis in my knee and there was nothing I could do about it. She sent me for more physiotherapy, but every exercise they gave me inflamed it more. I could not bend without pain. I could not even bear the weight of bedclothes on it.

During the Journey workshop I was so sure I hadn't done the process right that afterwards I was not watching for any changes that might occur. Then, I suddenly realized one day I had been squatting down for thirty minutes to do a job, putting a huge strain on my knee—and there was **no pain**.

A few days later, I walked half a mile downhill, briskly,

and realized at the bottom that I had not even thought of walking slowly and carefully.

It is wonderful to be able to dance, and walk to the village, and two weeks ago I did a hill walk with eighty steps downhill—and I was completely okay. What Joy!!

The physical healing is, of course, wonderful, but even more important is the knowledge that I can influence every cell in my body.

Upon hearing Anita's story at the meeting, another person stood up. Bill said he'd taken the Journey one year earlier and had come with chronic depression. After the weekend, he was convinced that everyone else had had a huge breakthrough and he'd been the only one who hadn't.

Bill forgot his process and went about his life, and it didn't dawn on him until *several months later* that he no longer suffered from depression. He explained that the whole reason he came to the grad support meeting was he wanted to thank me in person for something he'd "kind of taken for granted."

It is true—when we come into our natural state, it just seems so natural that we forget that it ever was any other way.

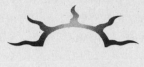

21

Some time ago I had a similar experience. Like my graduates, I too continue to get Journeywork done on myself when a physical or emotional issue arises. I noticed my vision was getting blurred. I had always enjoyed 20/20 vision, but as I was driving in my car I noticed that I was a little carsick. I saw a road sign in the distance that I would normally be able to read clearly, but it looked fuzzy and out of focus. I put it down to feeling a little tired and didn't think much more about it until the next day, when it happened again. After a week of blurred vision, I decided I'd better do a Physical Journey and uncover the problem. Being forty-three at the time, I knew that most people would say that this was the normal age when eyesight starts to deteriorate but I thought, "That's *not* my belief system. I don't believe it's an age thing. There must be something I'm somehow not willing to look at."

When I Journeyed inside the body, surprisingly I didn't end up where I thought I would. I just assumed I would end up inside my eyes and discover the problem there. Instead, when I got in my space shuttle, the infinite intelligence took me to my uterus. Although it didn't make any logical sense, I had learned from previous experience that the body wisdom *knows* where *it* wants to go and I've never known it to be wrong. So I decided to trust it.

In my womb I uncovered an old memory that had bothered me over the years. Whenever I tried to recall this memory, I was unsuccessful—it was a pure blank. My father had taken his life when I was nineteen years old, and I had felt emotionally devastated by his death. At the time, I'm sure I appeared outwardly centered, strong, and brave. I focused on helping my family go through the funeral process. But inwardly, I felt numbed and uncomprehending—unable to allow myself to feel or express the pain I was feeling. I've heard since then that often when someone commits suicide, the immediate family members somehow feel responsible. So mixed in with the numbness that barely covered the despair and grief was a profound sense of guilt—as if I should have been able to save him somehow.

After the funeral I went back to university and felt I was existing in an unreal world. I was a first-term student and had come to this new, strange, and lonely place only two weeks before my dad took his life. I felt alone, bereft, abandoned and cold, without a single friend to turn to.

In the memory I uncovered, it was a harsh, bitterly cold autumn night in upstate New York. I decided to go on a date with some guy I had barely met—just to distract myself from the pain. I didn't tell him what had happened with my dad, and put on a false, bright air, trying to appear mature and "with it." We went to a bar and drank some cocktails. I was completely unaccustomed to alcohol and quickly became drunk. Unlike my usual practical self, that night I had a brazen, reckless, devil-may-care attitude. I thought, "What does it matter anyhow? Nothing makes sense anymore. It's all pointless." I drank heavily, without caution.

On the way back to the dormitories we stopped by the liquor store and bought a quart of gin. When I got back to the guy's room, I downed three-quarters of the bottle myself. I must have passed out because I'd never been able to recall what took place after that.

Two days later I found myself walking in the woods near campus. I was cold, damp, wearing the same clothes from that night and felt emotionally ravaged, washed out, and disoriented. I felt a deep disgust with myself combined with a feeling of "I don't care anyway." I didn't know how I'd got there in the woods. Blearily, I found my way over to my department at university where I discovered notices up all over the bulletin boards. Apparently they had been looking for me for two-and-a-half days. I'd lost two days of my life and I had never remembered them—until this Physical Journey process.

I think the memory of those two days was too painful to look at, and it had been easier for my other-than-conscious mind to just block it out. But I guess at age forty-three, my soul felt it was time to finally face what took place and see what really happened during those two days. During my Physical Journey process I began to see flashes and snatches of what had taken place during that time.

It wasn't pretty.

I could understand why it was I had unconsciously protected myself from it all those years. But I finally *did* face it and I went through some deep process work and extensive forgiveness work. In this case, more than anything, it was *myself* I had to forgive for treating my life so carelessly, dangerously, and callously. And for punishing myself for a guilt I couldn't quell. I was lucky I survived that amount of alcohol. But then again, maybe that was the point.

When the Physical Journey was finished I expected there to be an immediate change in my eyesight. After all, I'd finally "looked at" something that for all those years had been unseeable. Three days went by and still no change. My eyes were still blurred and I was still getting carsick.

"Hmm," I thought, "how odd. It only takes forty-eight hours for the eye cells to replicate. Perhaps the infinite wisdom was wrong this time—perhaps I should have gone to my eyes instead of my womb." I forgot about the process and went on with my life. I made a pledge to myself that next time I did a Physical Journey, I would specifically choose to go to the eyes.

Three weeks later I came home late one night. The lights were not on in my garden and I suddenly noticed that my vision was so clear, I could see like an animal. I was keenly, sharply aware, able to see clearly in the dark. I could see the blades of grass and leaves—my night vision was sharper than I ever remembered.

The next day I noticed I no longer had carsickness. My vision had become clear again—it had crept up on me unawares, and I hadn't even noticed. It was so natural that I didn't even think about it. I was just like Anita and Bill, who hadn't noticed their own progress until after the fact.

I find that Journeywork is often like this. Once we're healed it's hard to conceive that we were any way other than healthy, normal, and natural. I find I have to remind people who do Journeywork to make sure that they keep score and take stock. In our neurology, success breeds success. And so, looking back at where we've come from and keeping score can be an important part of reinforcing healing.

I've noticed that sometimes with Journey process work it may take some time before the healing is complete. With each process, it's up to the inner intelligence to take each of us, uniquely, at a pace that is natural. Often it can seem like turning a switch off, and the old pattern is completely gone, instantly. But, at other times, it can feel more like a fan winding down. Have you ever switched off a fan, and noticed it takes some time for it to slow down and come to a full stop? With the Journey processes, it can sometimes be like that. Each time it is unique to the particular issue. There is no "right" time for healing.

So, would *you* like to undergo the same Physical Journey process that is used in my seminars? Once again, ask a friend you trust—preferably one who has already read this book—to set aside two hours to work with you. Make certain the time will be quiet and completely uninterrupted by noise or distraction of any kind.

You might like to read through the script a couple of times, just to become familiar with it. Then, when you're ready, you can begin. It's good to treat the script like an inner adventure—with the openness of a child. You can turn to the "Tools" section at the back of this book for the full Physical Journey process. It's very important to read the full instructions first.

22

Now that you've had the chance to undergo both the Emotional Journey and the Physical Journey, you might enjoy hearing some of the unexpected positive "side effects" of doing Journeywork.

Very often people have such a profound experience of Source that they find many old habits and limiting beliefs drop away spontaneously without them consciously working at it. The more they get in touch with their true self, the more the old, destructive patterns become obsolete and unnatural. Recently I have had several grads at the workshops speak of this phenomenon.

Noreen is a gregarious and warmhearted fifty-year-old Irish woman who counted herself very blessed to be the nanny to the children of two Journey grads. It happened by chance (or perhaps by destiny) that Noreen was asked to mind the children while the parents, Jerry and Cathy, attended the Abundance Retreat—a retreat that frees us from the many hidden ways we limit ourselves and unconsciously prevent ourselves from achieving abundance in our lives.

Noreen would sit outside the seminar room door in England patiently waiting for Cathy to come out during breaks to breastfeed her son. Soon everyone coming out of the room would find themselves sitting and chatting, regaled by Noreen's fiery wit and Irish charm. She, in turn, began to notice that there was something "special" about the people taking the seminar—a presence of love that seemed to emanate from them when she spoke to them. She noticed a certain sparkle—a twinkle in their eyes. She felt she really wanted to have some of whatever it was she experienced in everyone's presence, and decided there and then that she just *had* to take the Journey weekend seminar.

Noreen had suffered for years from chronic acute back pain, and had been diagnosed with a benign lump in her breast. She was interested in the possibility of healing herself, but more important, her *real* thirst was to find out what the "energy" was that she felt whenever she met someone from the seminar who was "awake" to their true self.

Noreen found her way to the very next Journey weekend workshop. She had a huge Emotional Journey process, and when she dropped through the layers and came into the experience of her own soul, her Source, it was so powerful that she made a decision to honor it at any cost.

Noreen felt that she had spent the whole of her life looking for this inner greatness—seeking this love that is in the core of us all. Once she had experienced the beauty in her own heart, she made a vow to be true to it, to be true to the diamond she had unearthed. She didn't want to do anything that would cover, stain, or sully this immense radiance; she just wanted to remain in the presence of it—to be in its simplicity and its purity and not leave it.

Noreen had always been a staunch drinking girl. It seemed like part of her Irish heritage. She went to the pub most nights, carousing with the girls, smoking and drinking, having a grand old time, often until the wee hours of the morning. She said to me she didn't really know any other life. "That's what people do, isn't it? You come home from work, have some food, and then it's off to the pub to enjoy a night out with your friends."

After taking the Journey she felt so completely at peace within— so content—that she found she didn't require constant activity or socializing to fulfill herself. The contentment was there all the time, whether she was working or playing. She felt so at peace with herself that at night she no longer felt compelled to burn the midnight oil, but began to revel in her own good company.

After some time, she said that the pubs began to feel too smoky and dark, and all interest in going to them fell away. Unexpectedly, she found that she was repulsed by cigarettes—they made her feel dirty and began to taste like sawdust—and, surprisingly, she didn't need the drink either—it began to taste like urine. She'd always found smoking and drinking relaxing, but now she felt *naturally* relaxed and had no need for them. To her surprise she began to crave more vibrant foods—wanting to eat more healthily. When she tried to eat meat she found she couldn't swallow it. And in time she became a vegetarian.

All this and yet there was *no effort* in it. All the old habits dropped away spontaneously once she recognized that *she* was this that she had been seeking. Once she felt true fulfillment and peace, she no longer wanted or needed old destructive habits that had always been a means to fill a deep emptiness inside.

She said she felt she had found a light inside that she wanted to honor and protect, and she truly understood what is meant when people say the body is the temple for the soul. That the lump in her breast and the chronic acute back pain also left her seemed almost incidental compared to this greater realization. She had discovered a precious diamond that she was no longer willing to cover.

Suzy was yet another Journey grad, who laughingly shared with me, "Brandon, I always thought those healthy people were so boring—you know the type, they drink Perrier, eat rabbit food, work out, don't smoke or drink booze—I always thought, 'They are all such goody-two-shoes. I don't want to be like them.' Now look at me, I've turned into one of them! I don't know what happened to me, but ever since the No Ego Retreat (an advanced level residential retreat) I really feel, for the first time in my life, I want to take care of my body. I actually care about myself and want to look after myself in the same way I would naturally care for someone I love."

As she spoke these words, I smiled, looking into her healthy vibrant eyes—amazed once again how the soul wants to cooperate with us in experiencing our own freedom—it really wants the highest and best for us.

Once you come to experience your own inner light, you start to cherish it and become less and less willing to do anything that might cover or obscure it. We become less willing to put a "lampshade" over our light. Marianne Williamson wrote about this so eloquently in her book *A Return to Love:*

Our deepest fear is not that we are inadequate. Our deepest fear is that we are powerful beyond measure. It is our light, not our darkness that most frightens us. We ask ourselves, "Who am I to be brilliant, gorgeous, talented, fabulous?" Actually, who are you not to be?

You are a child of God. Your playing small doesn't serve the world. There's nothing enlightened about shrinking so that people won't feel insecure around you. We are meant to shine, as children do. We were born to make manifest the glory of God that is within us. It's not just in some of us: it's in everyone. And as we let our own light shine, we unconsciously give other people permission to do the same. As we're liberated from our own fear, our presence automatically liberates others.

23

Our light is not the only thing we put a lampshade over. Very often we try to cover up and obscure our emotional feelings as well. I've found that this is especially true with addictions. Addictions can often be a means of distracting ourselves, or "putting a lampshade over" a deep emotional issue that we don't feel we can cope with or even face.

In our culture, we are often taught to address the SURFACE BEHAVIOR of an addiction (overeating, alcohol or drug addiction, compulsive shopping, stealing, or gambling, etc.), and yet we don't think to look at the CORE ISSUE of what is *causing* the behavior in the first place!

For instance, we may be aware that we have a challenge with our weight, and so we go about addressing it by changing our diet, going on fasts, or changing our exercise program. We address our *behavior*, but we don't think to ask, "Yes, but *why* am I overeating to begin with?"

So often we are successful with the new diet for only a short period of time, and then, slowly, our old ways creep back in and our weight increases once again. Why? Because we never found out what was *causing* us to overeat in the first place. The emotional root cause is still lurking inside the body, unaddressed.

Very often, at the Journey seminars, someone will raise their hand and say, "I don't have an emotional issue, my problem is that

I can't stop myself from overeating or snacking." Whenever someone says this I wonder what feeling they are trying to "stuff back down," what they have not yet been able to face. Of course they are not aware that they have an emotional issue—they've stuffed it down and put it to sleep *before* they've even given themselves a chance to feel what is really there.

We often hear the expression "comfort food." Well, what emotional feeling or issue needs comforting? The food numbs our ability to feel. How many of us can honestly say that we eat purely because the body is hungry and in need of nourishment?

So, in the seminar room, I often invite everyone to try this experiment. Just close your eyes. . . . Now imagine a recent time when you've reached for that snack food . . . a specific time . . . Once you've got the memory, roll the cameras back a few seconds to the very moment the impulse to grab for the food came up . . . (I wait for them to recognize it) . . . Now go back a few seconds *right before the impulse arose.* . . . Just before there is the decision to take action to get or eat the food, what are you *really* feeling? . . . Be willing to feel what is really there.

Inevitably, a look of surprise crosses everyone's face as they discover what it is they are actually feeling *before* the impulse arises, *before* they've escaped feeling it by stuffing it back down. Often it is a feeling of deep emptiness, loneliness, despair, or overwhelming anxiety. It is usually a *very strong and deep* emotion. As soon as we get a "whiff" of it, we are already reaching for the food to avoid it, run away from it, and put it back to sleep.

In Journeywork, I always say, "Wake up." Once you've identified the emotional issue that you're avoiding feeling, then you have the tools to finally deal with it in the Emotional Journey process! But if you're too busy stuffing it down, how will you ever get to the root cause and resolve it?

At a Journey workshop in London, one woman in her thirties with this exact problem raised her hand. She was clearly quite obese, and said she had been struggling with diets all her life. She really longed to be finished with it. When I asked her to do the process, she uncovered a deep feeling of shame mixed with fear. She opened her eyes completely stunned, and said she had *no idea* where that could have come from. She wasn't consciously aware of anything she was ashamed and fearful about. She really was puzzled. I suggested that she just trust that the emotional feeling was there for some reason, and that she use it as her starting point when she underwent her Emotional Journey process later that day.

When she was processing, I noticed that it appeared as if she'd uncovered something deeply upsetting. And, toward the end of her process, I could visibly see enormous relief in her entire body. As everyone's process is always kept private, I did not inquire what she had undergone, but I could tell it was big.

One month later, she came to our monthly grad meeting. She'd lost 26 pounds! With great enthusiasm she was the first one to raise her hand to share her success story. She said that, previously, she had never been able to remember anything before the age of ten—that somehow it was always a blank to her. During the Emotional Journey process, she finally got access to an earlier childhood memory that she'd not previously been able to recall. It was a childhood sexual abuse issue, which had been extremely traumatic, and she guessed she'd unconsciously blocked it out.

In her campfire process, not only did she finally access it, but, more important, she completely *resolved* it. Though she could never condone or forgive the *behavior* of the man involved, she said she wholeheartedly could forgive his *soul*. She said she'd felt free and so at ease ever since. The last I heard, she was continuing to lose weight.

Yet another man was at the Journey, and his problem was alcohol. He said he wouldn't call himself an alcoholic, but it was his common practice to have three or four pints of beer every night. When he went through the discovery process, he opened his eyes and meekly said, "I have fear of failure. I see my whole pattern. This fear arises when I sit at home and begin to relax so, even though my mind tells me I shouldn't, I say, 'Oh, I'll just have one beer.' Then it turns out to be three or four. Of course, the next morning I wake up feeling hungover and ragged, and I go to work and my performance isn't very good. I actually 'fail' at achieving the results I want. So, what do I do? Feeling bad about having been a failure, I go back home at night and drink more booze to numb myself to the fear. And so the cycle continues."

In his process, he uncovered childhood memories of being told by his dad that he would never amount to anything—he'd always be a failure. It had been a battle ever since then. The next time I saw him, his beer belly had disappeared, and he was glowing. He'd stopped drinking *and* smoking, and had succeeded in getting a better job.

These are only two people out of tens of thousands who have freed themselves from addictions by addressing the emotional cause, instead of solely going after the symptom. The Emotional Journey process was their key to freedom. They successfully uncovered the freedom and wholeness already waiting inside us all.

24

It seems it doesn't matter how old or young any of us is. There is a way in which we all have a sense that there is something large and free inside us. We have a knowing that we are capable of greatness and, secretly, we long to tap into our true potential and let it be fully expressed.

Noreen was sitting across the table from a former Catholic monk, an eighty-seven-year-old Irishman, having tea and a chat. He explained to her that, as he was getting older, he found it somehow comforting to sit quietly at the back of the local church—he felt such a peace and contentment there. However, something had been bothering him of late. Over the past few weeks, when the contentment arose, he found fear was emerging alongside it. He admitted to Noreen that it was making him feel reluctant to go to church for his daily contemplation.

Noreen asked, "What are you afraid of, Arthur?"

He flushed and answered in a broken whisper, "Dying . . . I think . . ." His voice trailed off.

Gently and simply, Noreen said, "Come with me to the sitting room, Arthur. Let me do a short process with you."

The old monk quietly followed Noreen, and settled down in an easy chair. Softly, Noreen guided him down through the emotional layers. When he dropped through the blackness into "peace," tears sprang to his eyes, and gently streamed down his cheeks. He opened his eyes and tenderly whispered, "Why don't they teach us this in the churches? All those years, and I never *knew*."

No matter what our age, each of us longs to remember who we truly are. Each of us longs to finally come "home." Going down through the layers is not the only way to tap into and directly experience the peace and freedom that is your Source. There are so many other ways that can take place in every moment of your daily life.

My experience is, once you've had a full awakening to this that you really are, Source keeps nagging you. It just won't leave you alone! Once you've journeyed home, home keeps beckoning you again and again. Truth keeps calling you into itself, until finally you fall so in love with it that you're not willing to do anything that would take you away from it.

On the second day of the Journey workshop, after everyone has already had a direct experience of dropping down through the layers and coming into Source, we begin to explore other more immediate and instantaneous ways of tapping into our inner awareness.

I always recommend going down through the layers as the first, most powerful option. Then, once you've experienced Source—even if all you did was "dip your toe in"—all the other myriad ways can be quite accessible.

One extremely powerful process is so simple that people are constantly amazed at how profound their experience of Source is, especially as this process is so very easy to do. It is an ancient process of self-inquiry that's been practiced for thousands of years in many Vedantan and Tibetan Buddhist monasteries. If you'd like, you can try it at home right now. It's best done with a partner.

Once again, set aside about one hour of private, quiet, uninterrupted time. Ask a friend—preferably one who has read this book—to sit down beside you. When you are both comfortable and ready you can close your eyes. Your friend will be asking a very simple question, and you are simply going to be relaxed and open like a child, really *longing* to know the answer—trusting that the answer may come in words, or as a word*less* response.

It's best if your friend really rivets their full attention to you, listening to you as if listening to the words of God. In this way, they are fully present to your experience, and they create a "sacred space" for you to begin your process.

Your friend will keep their eyes open, while yours are closed. They will begin by quietly asking, "Who are you?" With your eyes closed, resting in your own awareness, just tune in and allow the answer to bubble up from inside, without censoring anything that arises. Then, give your response out loud.

Your partner will then say, "Thank you," and ask you again, "Who are you?" Once again, just being relaxed, paying close attention to what's arising inside, respond out loud. Your partner will say, "Thank you," and ask, "Who are you?" once again.

And so you will continue in just this way.

Very often, at first, we may start by naming our surface roles: "I'm a teacher, mother, businessman, etc.," but if there is real openness and longing to know who you *really* are, then usually during the process, your deeper self will begin to reveal itself.

It may happen that at some point you feel yourself to be so vast, expansive, and silent that when "Who are you?" is asked, no actual words arise from within. If this happens, just be true to your experience, and be still.

Your partner will *still* say, "Thank you" to your *nonverbal response,* and once again ask, "Who are you?"

Your partner continues asking the question, waiting for your verbal or nonverbal reply and saying "Thank you," until the process is finished—in approximately fifteen to twenty minutes. Then you can stop, thank your partner, and switch roles.

The key to this exercise is to be open like a child, trust the very first words that come up, and be willing to share honestly, verbally, whatever does arise—no matter how ridiculous it may seem.

Some responses may not reveal their true meaning until later on, or they may even seem silly at the time. At one Journey seminar, I walked by a couple working together and heard one partner ask, "Who are you?" The other partner answered, "I'm a gas pump." The first partner half smiled and said, "Thank you . . . Who are you?"

I didn't hear the rest of their process, until the one who had experienced himself as a gas pump revealed that he had realized that not only was he the gas pump, but also the gas, the gas station, the air, and finally that he was *everything*. He felt himself to be *all of life*, and also that all of life was happening *in him*—including the gas pump!

So, no matter how silly it may sound, please don't censor yourself. Let Source reveal its nature in its own magical and mysterious ways. It's a simple exercise, but extremely profound. For me, it is my favorite.

I like to take a few minutes out of my busy day just to sit quietly, go within and inquire "Who am I?" Usually, I can barely get through this sentence before the vast, powerful realization of myself in everything, everywhere reveals itself. I rest in a thought-free wordless presence of stillness that is so awe-inspiring that it often brings tears to my eyes, and I recognize it to be who I am.

Very often, in the "Who are you?" process, it is as powerful to be the listener, riveting your attention to your partner, as it is to be asked, "Who are you?" This simple, powerful principle is something you can easily apply in your everyday life. Just allow your whole being to be focused on whatever task you are doing. If you really rivet your attention, if you are completely present, then you may experience the timeless awareness that is always present when no thought occurs. You'll find yourself living moment-to-moment as a never-ending stream of nowness—present awareness. In it there is pure simplicity, thought-free stillness, and absolute fearlessness (the absence of fear). In this awareness, action takes place quite gracefully, freely and efficiently—when there are no thoughts distracting you, or pulling you off course. Awareness is not disturbed by action, and is actually the wellspring from which all genius and inspiration comes.

Still another way to directly experience the Self is through meditation. Many of you who are reading this book may have learned specific "methods" of meditation. I am not referring to the kind of meditation where you focus your mind on a word or a mantra. Nor am I speaking about the type of meditation where you direct your mind to the various sensations in the body. Very often, I think, people who practice meditation mistake a trancelike state for the freedom that I'm referring to. What I'm speaking about is not sleepy in the slightest. It is not detached, zoned-out, mellowed-out, numbed-out, or zombielike. It is the quintessence of wakefulness. It is keen, sharp, present, and scintillating with aliveness. It is crystal clear, pure beingness, and in it you feel connected with everything. In fact, you know you *are* everything.

Often I have heard it said that meditation is a time for contemplating and reviewing your thoughts. For many it is a time when the mind runs riot, jumping around like a bunch of chattering monkeys. So, if you have a specific method, please do not mistake it for what I am speaking about here.

I have been meditating for over twenty-five years, and though I found it relaxing and quieting, meditation as it is commonly taught did not cause me to "wake up," or give me the full realization of who I am. This peace I'm referring to is a stillness *beyond* the mind. In it is an energy, a power of love that will often give rise to a causeless joy. The type of meditation I am speaking about I prefer to call "sitting." It is a resting, steeping, soaking in awareness itself, in stillness as pure beingness. No thoughts, no mantras, no methods. And I've found that just by asking, "Who am I?" this presence can reveal itself powerfully.

Would you like to try a "methodless" meditation? Would you like to experience "sitting"?

Set about twenty or thirty minutes aside. Find a comfortable position in which you can sit quietly by yourself. You can begin by asking, "Who am I?" Allow the full wordless presence to reveal itself. . . . Just soak in this presence.

If you like, you can allow that presence, that awareness to expand boundlessly in front of you. . . . Then feel it becoming vast behind you. . . . Then let it become spacious to all sides of you . . . endless below . . . and infinite above . . . and let yourself rest as a boundless sea of pure beingness, an ocean of stillness.

If thoughts come through, you can let them be like so much flotsam and jetsam drifting on the surface, as you remain deeply immersed in the presence of awareness.

Or, if thoughts pass through, let it be none of your business—treat them like so many clouds in the sky, just drifting by as you remain soaking, steeping in the depths of this fathomless sea of stillness, in pure awareness.

Just let yourself remain very vast, very boundless, soaking in this way until an inner knowing or impulse compels you to complete.

I like to let "sitting" in this way take as long as it likes, but at the minimum I always allow at least twenty minutes. When you open your eyes, keep your awareness very light, open, and spacious. Be aware of your presence filling the room, then all the action of your day can happen naturally in this vaster context. In fact, I find this presence has an innate intelligence that allows my whole day to take place fluidly. Resting in it, action happens effortlessly and gracefully without my getting in the way of things. In this awareness, so much more gets done without the normal striving and efforting.

25

In the Journey seminar, after the "Who are you?" process is complete, I ask everyone, "What are some of the qualities that seem to arise naturally out of Source?" People call out the various qualities, and the words are all put up onto a big whiteboard at the front of the room. The entire board gets filled with these beautiful qualities.

When you did your "Who are you?" process, what were some of the qualities that came up for you? Pictured below is a typical whiteboard.

Freedom, boundlessness, joy, clarity, abundance, forgiveness, synchronicity, awareness, peace, humor, fluidity, grace, stillness, fearlessness, openness, silence, divinity, surrender, beingness, alacrity, spontaneity, lightness, wisdom, care, compassion, effortlessness, beauty, trust, inspiration, healing, vitality, fun, laughter, purity, playfulness, excitement, fulfillment, serendipity, oneness, humility, understanding, acceptance, delight, honoring, strength, courage, vastness, aliveness, vibrancy, passion, balance, timelessness, gentleness, curiosity, simplicity, pure energy, tenderness, wholeness, completeness, serenity, truth.

Once the whiteboard is filled, I ask everyone to look at the qualities and really imbibe them. And I ask how many of these qualities
they have experienced during the weekend. There is usually a
long pause, as people reflect on the question, and inevitably
someone pipes up and says, "Every one of them!"

I always answer that this is absolutely true. We have experienced every one of them. Any time Source wants you to know
you are in touch with it, it gives you a gift in the form of one of
these qualities. It's the way that your essence, your soul, has of
communicating in no uncertain terms that you are in touch with
your deepest Self. It's the way Source has of saying, "Right on!
You're in touch. And because you're in touch, you get the prize,
you get the gift!" You're in touch, so you get to feel joy, delight,
peace. It's the way awareness can signal to the body that you're on
track.

Every time you're in touch it leaves you a clue, and if you start
looking for the moments in your life when you have felt any one
of these qualities (compassion, tenderness, clarity, etc.), this is
Source signaling you that you are in flow.

So many people say, "I wish I knew what I'm supposed to do in
life." Well, look for the clues—Source is leaving you bread
crumbs all along the path. If you but follow the bread crumbs
from one experience of Source to the next, you can lead your life
as a never-ending flow of Source, following your soul's design for
your life rather than getting trapped by your conflicting ideations
and confusing mind-talk.

Your body is a barometer of the soul. If you want to know if you're
on track, check your body. If you are experiencing any of the
qualities of Source, give yourself a big pat on the back—you're in
touch, you're in flow.

In this way your soul can guide you from one experience of
Source to the next.

26

Not everyone who does Journey process work arrives with a challenging emotional issue or health problem. As a matter of fact, *most* of the people already have much of their lives well in order. They may already feel healthy, and lead successful and fulfilling lives.

I think a true sign of success is the honest recognition that there is *always* room for improvement, always more growing and learning to do. Success tends to breed more success, and to continue to succeed, you must grow. And so, highly successful people often come to The Journey for a general internal "house cleaning," to become even *more* free, *more* alive *and more* healthy, in their relationships, at work, or within themselves. They come to be more successful.

Often when people have achieved everything—the perfect family, the house in the country, and have highly successful jobs—something inside them says, "I've achieved everything *I thought* I wanted, and yet I just know there is *something more—* something greater."

These are the very people who often have the greatest longing to wake up to their true self, to Source. They've realized that all the outer trappings may be pleasant but they just "know it's not enough." It's "not IT." These people often become real spiritual seekers. Having sought the greatness in the outer world and having realized that there is something missing, they begin to turn their attention inward, hoping to find the truth that will set them free.

This thirst to come to know who you really are is to me the most profound thirst there is. A thirst of the highest order. Very often these seekers aren't even aware that this is what they are seeking. All they know is that there is *something* greater, and they want to experience it, to know it, to live in it.

Sometimes, it's only when you have all your ducks in a row, when everything seems to be going right, that your soul whispers to you, "Yes, *and* there's something more." It's then that people find themselves in private one-to-one sessions or at The Journey weekend.

I always believe that if people have made it to The Journey or picked up this book, it must mean that the soul is ready. Somewhere inside, they have put out a strong prayer—a prayer to wake up to the truth, a prayer to find the greatness within. I feel so honored, so humbled to meet the people who come for one-to-one sessions or are drawn to The Journey workshops, because I know that they have put out this divine prayer and that even if their conscious mind isn't aware of it, their soul is calling them home.

They've come to discover their *true selves* and if they are very lucky, they may fall so deeply in love with Source, with truth, that they decide they want never to leave it.

Geoffrey is one such man. He is the managing director of a highly successful company in Manchester, England. When he arrived for his one-to-one session he seemed self-assured, dynamic—a real achiever type. I would imagine that most people would consider his lifestyle to be enviable—he has a beautiful daughter, lovely wife, gorgeous home, and successful career. Virtually everything in his life appeared to be moving in the right direction.

He let me know that everything was actually going quite well and that he'd really only come to sort out some minor things, for some "fine tuning." It had been bothering him that, although he was the managing director of a successful computer firm, he still found he had a fear of public speaking and felt shy and awkward when making presentations in front of his board of directors. He explained how ridiculous this was, as the company was doing so well, and how foolish it made him feel to be the managing director and yet be so blatantly awkward in front of his own board. "I know I'm a good leader—our results indicate that—but when it comes to public speaking, I freeze."

We laughed and I explained that here in the United States they did a survey, and found out that fear of public speaking is actually the number one fear—greater than the fear of death! I went on to say that this awkwardness that he felt was extremely common. I said, "Since people fear public speaking more than death, you're probably well ahead of the game, because at least you're getting up there to deliver speeches. That's more than most people feel they are capable of doing."

He smiled but reiterated that he still longed to be free from anything that might be holding him back. I agreed and said that I had the same commitment in my life to go after any challenge that seems to hold me back on any level. Then I assured him that I would do my best to help him uncover what was at the bottom of this fear, so that he could finally set himself free from it.

Before we started his process work, he looked at his watch, and let me know he had a meeting to get to, a plane to catch and that it all needed to be completed and finished by 2 P.M. Basically, he had come to get rid of his greatest fear and he wanted it handled in an hour-and-a-half's time! Even when it came to personal growth he expected to achieve the best results in record time. I smiled and said I'd give it my best shot.

As I reached for my clipboard, silently I made the prayer I always make for clients before I start—that the highest and deepest healing take place on every level of his being—emotionally, physically, and spiritually. And in my heart I was reminded that although he thought he was there to cure himself of the fear of public speaking, in fact he was going to be getting so much more—he would come to know his true self—the infinite wisdom, the inner genius.

Though he'd not mentioned it, I knew that somewhere inside he'd put out a prayer to "wake up" to who he *really* is and that even though fear of public speaking was his surface emotional issue, his real longing was for freedom, for peace, for truth itself.

As we went down through the emotional layers, he gave a running commentary, as if he was keeping score of how well he was doing. Even in his process, his achiever identity was strongly coming through. For part of the process, I felt this commentary almost got in the way and I had to remind him to stay out of his head and just feel and be present to his emotions. Eventually he finally broke through. It was a humbling experience for us both. Here was this man sitting in his perfectly ironed shirt and silk tie, with tears of awe and wonder streaming down his cheeks—wonder at the awe-inspiring beauty he'd discovered, the vast, boundless oneness with everyone and everything. He sat silently, deeply moved by the powerful presence of love in his own heart.

Once he was in touch with his own infinite wisdom, it was quite extraordinary how clearly his childhood patterns were revealed. He saw scene after scene with his father in which he felt he would never be good enough for his dad. If he brought home an exam marked 95 out of 100, his father would say "What happened to the other 5 points?" It seemed that no matter how hard he tried, no matter how much he'd achieved, he'd never win his father's respect or approval.

He saw with absolute clarity what was at the core of this fear of public speaking. And how, even with his board of directors, he felt he'd never win their respect, no matter how much he'd achieved. It was almost as if, every time he stood up to speak in front of the board, he was actually a small boy standing before his father. The old fear of "I'll never get it right. I'll never be good enough" was causing him to crumble internally.

After he completed the process work and resolved the issue with his father, forgiving him for all the times he felt so misunderstood, unloved, and disapproved of, we continued going through the remaining emotional layers.

When we were done, I looked into the eyes of a man who had finally found peace. He looked like a young, innocent child. He glanced down at his watch and realized that he was just in time to catch his plane, but thought that maybe he'd cancel the board meeting that afternoon. He admitted that it was such a huge revelation for him that he wanted to take a few moments just to savor it and integrate it. Inwardly I noted what an unlikely response that would have been for the man who had walked through my door just two hours earlier.

Two weeks later, I was at a Journey seminar and surprisingly Geoffrey strolled into the seminar room. I hadn't actually expected him to come, because of his busy schedule, and I was delighted to see him.

At one point during a question and answer session, Geoffrey raised his hand and proudly and fearlessly stood up to speak in front of a room of over 100 people. He spoke eloquently and breezily and inspired everyone, as if speaking in public was as natural to him as tying his shoelaces.

"What an about-face," I thought. He shared that he had previously had a fear of public speaking and had come for a one-to-one session with me. Not only had the fear gone, but since then, he felt himself to be so in the flow, in the "zone," that his golf game had improved significantly. In fact, he *won* a golf tournament two days after the session.

Everyone applauded his obvious success. And then he added, "When I got up to receive my trophy I gave an acceptance speech flawlessly and easily. It was then that I realized my fear of public speaking had left me."

When he sat down, I looked into his eyes and saw that same twinkle—that sparkle that I so often see when someone has woken up and come home to their true self. He positively glowed. And I thought, "Isn't it amazing how even a businessman whose whole focus has been on achievement longs to know this inner love, this peace?"

For the first time he *truly* looked successful to me. He'd found that priceless treasure that no one could take from him. He'd found his real self.

Yet another man came to a workshop, but in his case almost the opposite had been true. In his forties, Alan had been a highly successful businessman, having made millions. Now in his sixties, he had lost his entire fortune and had to rely on a friend to pay his course fee for the weekend.

During his Physical Journey process he had an unexpected event take place. His space shuttle had taken him into his eye, which looked all cloudy from the inside, looking out. Interestingly, though, the memory he uncovered was not a negative memory from his past, but a *positive* one. Alan went back to a time in his life when he was highly successful—a real go-getting achiever and entrepreneur. He went back to a time when it seemed as if everything he touched turned to gold, a time when it seemed that nothing could stop him.

There were no other people at his campfire—just the younger forty-year-old Alan, the present-day Alan and his mentor. But, boy did the younger him have a lot to say! The younger Alan gave the present-day Alan a real talking to, reminding him in no uncertain terms that the same genius, the same positive qualities that had made him a millionaire in his forties, were still inside him. They were sitting there fallow and unused because the present-day Alan had forgotten who he was. He had forgotten the greatness that had allowed him to achieve such success. The younger him was upbraiding him, imploring him to recognize, "I'm still here!"

It hadn't occurred to the present-day Alan that his success hadn't been a product of outer circumstances. He hadn't realized that his success had been born out of his own inner greatness. It was the first time in over ten years that Alan even contemplated the possibility of succeeding again.

After the process, Alan said he felt he had a skip in his step, and that he felt truly freed from the helpless victim state that he'd been a prisoner of for so many years. It had taken the process for him to remember what it was to be in touch with Source again, and how it felt to tap into his own inner genius. It was the first time he felt in flow, in touch, in years. He hadn't thought it was possible.

When he got ready to leave the seminar, I saw a youthful twinkle in his eye that I'm certain must have been what he looked like in his successful younger days. He'd remembered the spark of being in touch with his real, free Self.

27

It's been my own personal experience that The Journey doesn't end with one Physical or Emotional Journey process. In fact, usually doing the process is just the *beginning* of a lifetime of letting go of emotional layers, and an ever-deepening experience of yourself in Freedom. Freedom has no boundaries. It's not like you arrive in Source and you are established in it. Rather, it's more like you start living in Source, as an expression of it, and it reveals all the remaining veils, wounded patterns, and old issues that are ready to be let go of. This that you truly are draws you more and more deeply into itself, yet it remains still, pristine and untouched by the whole dance of life.

Source is relentless in its desire to free you. By its very nature, Freedom calls to the surface anything that is not yet free, and says, "This is welcome, but it's not who you *really* are." Source has a way of pointing to this that you are *not,* even while taking you deeper into this that you truly *are.* So when the tumor came and left, I didn't realize that this would be just the beginning of a lifetime of letting go.

About one-and-a-half years after the tumor, in the fall of 1993, there was a big firestorm in the hills of Malibu. Perhaps you read about it in the newspaper or saw it on television. The fires were so devastating that they took 280 homes and left hundreds without a place to live.

I was in New York City at the time, in a television studio. The director came up to me and said, "I think you'd better leave the set and go to the green room lounge to watch the news. You have a home in Malibu, don't you? Perhaps you'd better make sure everything is all right. The reports are saying the fire is out of control, and the flames are over 70 feet high."

As I watched the news, none of it made sense—it seemed surreal. There was my hometown, beautiful Malibu, thick with black smoke and blazing like an inferno. Quietly, I sat alone in the lounge and watched as, one by one, friends' homes went up like so many matchsticks. It felt like a poorly edited disaster movie, and it seemed like soon the credits would start rolling.

I couldn't see my own house, but as the fires were clearly moving across the hillsides and my house was on the beach, it didn't seem as though there was much possibility that the flames would leap over the highway and set the beach houses on fire.

Feeling like I wasn't really helping matters by sitting there stunned and hypnotized in front of a television screen, I switched it off and decided to sit quietly and pray for all the people who suddenly had their lives turned inside out. I knew there must be so much suffering going on, and I thought of my friends and sent them all my love. Unable to reach them, I felt very alone and helpless. I so longed to be able to do anything at all, and praying was the best thing I could think of.

After the prayers were finished, I just sat there, quietly riveted in a timeless stillness with nothing to say or do. Softly, into the stillness, an inner foreboding began to arise. I decided I'd better do a quick mental checklist to make sure that none of my loved ones were in my house—just in case. I thought of my daughter, Kelley, and how she had recently moved eight miles away to Santa Monica with her fiancé. And I knew Don was in Santa Fe taking a seminar. We no longer had any pets so, for a moment, I felt a sigh of relief that none of my family was at home . . . and yet, quietly, that inner foreboding began to snake its way into my guts.

Shaking it off, I decided to call my daughter and her fiancé to make sure they were all right, and once that was all clear I asked the director to be allowed to leave early.

That night I slept fitfully and woke the next morning with a splitting migraine. I went straight to the studios. When I got there, everyone stopped to look at me. I thought I had arrived late. There was a terrible hush in what was otherwise a busy, chirpy crew.

Two people kept exchanging glances, as if to decide who was going to break the news to me. Finally, mercifully, someone wound up the nerve and said, "Brandon, I think you need to book your flight home. . . . Your house has just burned down. . . . Sorry . . . don't know what to say." Awkward pause . . . "Did you have insurance?"

"No . . . no one does in Malibu—it's just too expensive when you live by the sea . . ." Another long pause . . . "Well, I guess I'd better find out if the airlines can help me out." No one said anything else. There was nothing more that could be said.

I stepped outside the studio doors into the sharp, cold New York wind. It was a gray fall day, but the colors seemed keenly intense, the smells so strong, the traffic noise blaring, and yet in all of this I felt a very deep quiet.

Oddly, I felt as if some great burden had been lifted from my shoulders, as if years of karma had left me somehow. I felt curiously light and free. From inside, a little song I had heard at a spiritual center began to play itself. The words were, "Have faith, everything is all right." They seemed ridiculously corny, yet sweetly appropriate, so I continued to sing the tune to myself as I walked back to the hotel to pack my bags.

I called the airlines. Though I had a nonrefundable ticket, they agreed that under the circumstances I could fly standby, but warned me that the next flight was quite full. When I arrived at the airport the flight was fully booked, and as there were no more coach-class seats available, a very kind lady upgraded me to first class. Tears sprang to my eyes at the generous heart of a complete stranger so clearly reaching out to me at a time when I most needed it. The song "Have faith, everything is all right" continued to play inside my head.

On the flight home, I had an awareness that the clothes in my suitcase were the sum total of what I owned. Here I was, forty years old, and all I had was a suitcase to my name. Somehow, it didn't seem such a bad thing.

On arriving at Los Angeles airport, my husband greeted me and said, "I think it would be best if we went straight there. You have your driver's license with you, don't you? They're not letting anyone through the barricades unless you can prove you are a resident whose house has burned down. Each person has to show proof. Already there's been so much looting."

As we drove up the Pacific Coast Highway, it no longer looked like a surreal disaster movie. Everything was very, very real. The devastation took my breath away. When we got close to what used to be our home, I took in a deep breath to prepare myself. Yet nothing could truly prepare me. When we pulled into the driveway, all that was left was black and burned timber, still steaming in places, a lot of rubble, and our magnificent magenta-colored bougainvillea—still untouched, fresh, in full bloom, looking so vibrant and alive in contrast to the stark black pile of what was the remains of eighteen years of family life.

I had expected to burst into tears, but instead I felt deeply quiet, humbled, and aware that this was a sacred moment for me—a precious moment. I didn't want to suppress or obscure anything that I might feel. I just wanted to be present to whatever might come up. A deep, unexplainable feeling of gratitude came washing through me. I became aware of how lucky I was to have such a loving relationship with my husband and daughter, and this was, after all, all that really mattered. Everything else was just material "stuff."

As we stepped into what would have been our kitchen, Don cautioned me to be careful, as the floors had burned through. A few pieces of blackened wood remained standing, the fridge and dishwasher had completely melted, and the plastic had fused to the metal. I could see the signs that whatever pottery hadn't fallen and smashed had already been looted. It seemed somehow bizarrely ludicrous that people would actually prey upon someone else's loss and steal from those who already had next-to-nothing left.

Nothing about the remains seemed to resemble what I had come to know of as our home until I came across a piece of pottery that the looters had missed. It was a mug that I bought at that spiritual center. On it were written the simple words, "Have faith, everything is all right." I laughed to myself, and realized I was being left signs that Grace was definitely at hand.

Don and I continued to dig through the rubble, to see if there might be the occasional keepsake or piece of memorabilia that might be worth salvaging. Amazingly, a metal filing cabinet had fallen on our heavy leather-bound wedding album. We were thrilled to find it, and though the pictures were partially soaked with water, they still were intact. I also came across a badly marred metal button that a teacher had once given me. On it were written the words, "When life gives you lemons, make lemonade." It seemed like I was being left signs everywhere, and I smiled at the thought of just how much lemonade I'd probably be making.

Each moment seemed both precious and poignant, not at all as I had thought it would be. We laughed at how much better the view of the ocean was, now that there were no walls, and continued digging our way through the remains. Suddenly, and unexpectedly, I heard a voice behind me. I turned around and found myself face to face with a huge television camera. A reporter jammed a microphone under my mouth and asked, "Do you mind if I ask you a few questions?" Startled and stunned, I mumbled, ". . . Well, no . . . as long as you don't mind me getting on with the work. . . . We've just arrived here."

"Well, how does it feel to be a victim of this disaster?"

Shaking my head incredulously, at the amazing insensitivity of asking a question like that at a time like this, I nonetheless softly replied, "Well, actually, I don't feel myself to be a victim."

"Okay, so how does it feel to be a *survivor* of this disaster?"

I looked at her and quietly said, "Well, actually I don't feel myself to be a survivor, either."

"Okay, so how *do* you feel?" Finally she'd asked the first *real* question.

"Well, truthfully, what I'm feeling most right now is gratitude."

"Gratitude? How could you feel gratitude at a time like this?"

Finally, I stopped digging around. I turned and looked straight into her eyes. It flashed through my mind as I saw her face how difficult it must be to be a reporter. Quietly, I said, "I feel gratitude because I am truly aware today of how most people would gladly burn down ten houses to experience the kind of love that I have in my life—to have the deeply fulfilling relationship I have with my husband, and to feel how blessed I am to be so close with my daughter."

Pointing at the rubble, I said, "This is not a disaster. If you're looking for a disaster, go speak to the eighty-year-old woman who lived at the top of that hill. She never sees her children anymore, and her house was all she had left. Now that's a disaster. Me, I'm forty years old. I have people I love and a career I feel privileged to work in. You wouldn't say to an eighteen-year-old, 'Oh, what a disaster—you have nothing but two suitcases in your hands to start up life with.' You'd say, 'You have your whole life ahead of you.' I'm like that teenager. I may be forty years old, and no, I don't have any insurance, but I have my whole life ahead of me. So, no, this is not a disaster."

She asked the cameraman to cut, and privately asked me if I *really* felt this way. She had tears in her eyes. Quietly I answered, "You know, at a time like this it doesn't occur to you to make something like that up. There is a lot of vulnerability and humility at a time like this, and truth has a way of speaking itself plainly."

"But how could you feel grateful, when you know your house is the *only* beach house that went up in flames? Doesn't that make you feel, 'Why me? Why my house?' " I saw her signal the cameraman to start rolling again.

"Well, let me tell you the real story of this house. Ten minutes before you walked in, I spoke to a fireman, who said he was here at the time of the fire. An ember had flown across the highway, and though an entire fire squad was poised outside my house, ready to douse the flames, they couldn't stop it because the seventy-mile-an-hour winds were too strong. It was out of their control. So the house burned down to the ground in less than five minutes. He also told me something much more interesting. He said the whole house burned down except this one room over here—my meditation room. He said, 'I don't know what it was about that room, but the fire stopped there.' They were able to douse out the rest of the flames.

"Because of that one mysterious room, all the neighboring beach cottages were saved. So, if my house had to be sacrificed so that all the others could be saved, well then, that is a small price when you look at the whole picture."

With this last answer the reporter seemed at a loss for words, and having run out of questions, she and the cameraman quietly packed up and left.

The fireman stopped by later, and asked what it was about that room that made it so special. He seemed genuinely perplexed. None of his colleagues on the fire team could figure it out.

"Well," I said, "I recently had this room built onto the deck. Because it was my meditation room, I put pictures of saints from various spiritual traditions inside the walls as it was being built. Now, I can't explain the mystery of why it didn't burn down, but if the fire stopped there, all I can suggest is perhaps there was some protective Grace in it somehow. I can't really give you an answer, but the important thing is our neighbor's house, which is butted up next to it, remained completely untouched by flames. And for that I do feel grateful."

"Well, if it had reached your neighbor's house, the fire would have taken every house on this strip of Malibu beach, because there was no way we could have stopped it."

Shaking his head, he added, "I don't believe in those kind of things, but as a fireman, I know my business—and it does make you wonder."

It didn't make me wonder. It seemed the signs of Grace were all over the place. And truly, I was left with everything that really mattered—my husband, my daughter, and my ability to earn enough money to put food in our bellies and, eventually, a roof over our heads. Most of all, I was left feeling abundant—like I was blessed with what really mattered in life, love itself. Or, at least so it seemed at the time.

28

Life had something deeper to teach me about the true nature of love.

It was a year after the fire. We had settled into a new apartment in Malibu, south of all the devastation; this time in the hills with a view of the ocean. Somehow Grace seemed to be supporting us in getting our lives started again from scratch. So many people, even complete strangers, were kind and generous to us during that year. Furnishing our new home had taken every dime we had, and so Don had written several letters to the Internal Revenue Service requesting that, under the circumstances, we be put on a payment plan to pay our overdue taxes. The fire had been financially devastating, and we were doing what we could to get our lives back together.

Don and I had been working out of the country for nearly two months. Our air tickets allowed a stopover in India, and so, on a shoestring and a prayer, we went to visit a spiritual teacher there. It seemed it was time for so many lessons—first the tumor, then the fire, and when we visited the teacher I felt a deep surrender and an unslakable thirst to learn whatever Source had to teach of its nature.

During our stay, I had a crashing spiritual experience—a feeling that my "pot had been smashed"—that my own separate identity, all that I thought was "me," my ego, had crumbled into dust.

What was left was pure awareness shining in everything, everywhere. On the plane ride home, there was the awareness that I was looking at everything with fresh eyes, as if for the first time. Everything was scintillating *as* me. I had no idea that what lay ahead in Malibu would end up mirroring the experience in India. My life would never be the same.

Lugging my heavy suitcases up the stairs to our new apartment, weary and tired from the long trip, I still found myself seeing everything freshly. The jade tree looked so lush. The flowering ice plant looked so vibrant. And when I stepped into the apartment, threw open our sliding glass doors, and drank in the fresh sea air, filling my lungs with the salty-seaweed smell of the ocean, I wondered if it had ever smelled this glorious.

I looked behind me at the kitchen table. There was a stack of mail piled high, which had always given me a "welcome—yes, you've arrived home" feeling. So, before unpacking our bags, I rifled quickly through the pile, to see if perhaps there was some good news from someone. Five heavily stuffed envelopes, addressed from the IRS, and dated at different times were among the other letters. "Great," I thought, "they must have finally responded to Don and put us on a payment plan." Though I usually left the bills for Don, I felt strangely compelled to open them first.

Expecting good news, I was not prepared for what I read. Shocked, I thought, "There must be some mistake. Can they really do this? We've just been devastated by the fire." Thinking it must be a mistake, I quickly tore open another, more recent IRS letter. Same words, only more demanding. They were taking *one hundred percent* of our wages and were freezing our bank accounts.

"How is it possible that, when you have lost everything in a fire, the government could take away even your ability to put food on a table? Didn't they realize they were taking *everything* we had?" I felt the wind had been knocked out of me.

"Don, you need to look at these."

I stood at the kitchen table stunned, unable to think. Looking for something that might be a little more friendly to read, I tore through the pile, and found a letter from my daughter, Kelley. Kel had always been my soul mate. I prided myself on the deep abiding respect we had for one another—how we could tell each other anything, and shared our deepest secrets. I felt ours was not just a special mother-daughter relationship, but a remarkable one. Her handwriting instantly warmed my heart, and I made a mess of opening the envelope, not able to open it quickly enough.

My heart stopped. Tears flashed to my eyes. Her words cut through me. She wrote that while we were away, she had been through some dramatic life changes, and on looking back through her life she felt Don and I had been too strong an influence on her. She really didn't want to have any more contact with us, and didn't know when she would. She left no number, and no forwarding address.

Her letter had come so out of the blue—seemingly out of nowhere. I truly couldn't imagine what we had done or said—it just didn't make sense. We'd just arrived home, and in five minutes it seemed as if our whole world was coming tumbling down around us.

Two days later, not knowing where to turn, with no money to pay a lawyer to help us, and not having a clue about who else to ask about the IRS, Don and I were standing in our bedroom. There was a feeling in the air of everything being on tenterhooks, on shaky ground. Under the strain, Don's temper seemed to flare, and unexpectedly he blurted out that I needed to "get real" and wake up to what was going on around me—and not just with the finances. Didn't I know that he had fallen in love with another woman? Hadn't I figured it out yet?

I stood there openmouthed, absolutely stunned. Eventually, thinking he might have a crush on someone we both knew, I mumbled, "Who? . . . What do you mean 'in love with another woman'? . . . Who is it?"

"It's someone I met on my fiftieth birthday, last August. We've been passionately in love ever since."

Still stunned and uncomprehending, I stupidly asked, "Are you physically involved?"

He gave me a "Must I spell it out to you?" look, and said, "What did you think I meant by 'passionately'? This is not some one-night thing, Brandon. This is serious. I've already spoken to her about marriage."

I was dumbstruck, blown out of the water. I'd never seen any signs or clues of anything. I was so unsuspecting, so trusting. We were both so much in love with each other. Our marriage seemed so alive. It wasn't as if we had a dead, empty marriage like so many I'd seen. We both still called each other our "true love," and Don still had the ability to make my heart skip when I heard his car pull up. Ours had been a high romance, a "legendary love." Even the spiritual teacher in India had commented on the rarity of the devotion we had for each other, and how we were an extraordinary example to all couples. I'd always seen us holding hands, together in rocking chairs, still deeply in love with one another until we died.

It was the only thing in life I was absolutely certain of. Don and Brandon were two names set together in stone. This must be some mistake. The words just didn't match what I knew in my heart to be true. The words didn't match what I knew was the reality—that he loved me more than life itself, as I did him.

The conversation went on into the mundane particulars, as he pointed out to me all the signs I stupidly and trustingly had missed. As I walked out into the living room, it seemed as if the whole world as I knew it came crashing in around me. Nothing was as it seemed. Nothing was certain or real anymore. Everything I had thought of as my life had been stripped away, and there was nothing to cling to, nowhere to turn. It felt like free-falling—free-falling in nothingness. No walls to grab onto, and nowhere to land.

The tumor, the fire, the IRS, no money, husband leaving,

daughter gone—was there anything else that I had thought was my life that could go? It was just like in India, when I felt my ego had been smashed. Here my identity in the world as I knew it— mother, beloved wife, livelihood, even my ability to survive— had been stripped away. Was there nothing certain or permanent in the world?

Feeling extremely present and sharply aware, I walked up the stairs to the kitchen to get a glass of water. As I passed the refrigerator door, a quote our dear friend Robbie had given us strongly caught my eye. The words arrested me. They seemed to leap off the page—"Know whatever comes to you unexpected to be a gift from God, which will surely serve you if you use it to the fullest. It is only that which you strive for out of your own imagination, that gives you trouble." I read it three times. The words penetrated me to the core.

"KNOW WHATEVER COMES TO YOU *UNEXPECTED* TO BE A GIFT FROM GOD, WHICH WILL SURELY SERVE YOU IF YOU USE IT TO THE FULLEST. IT IS ONLY THAT WHICH YOU STRIVE FOR OUT OF YOUR OWN IMAGINATION, THAT GIVES YOU TROUBLE."

As I stared at them, I knew them to be true. Every cell in my body knew they were true. Truth itself knew that Truth was speaking. And though I couldn't know the mystery of what was happening, all I could really do was trust that somehow there would be a gift in it, and that if I used it fully it would surely serve me.

Once again, in the middle of catastrophe, the signs of Grace were speaking loud and clear. Time stood still. All fell silent, and a profound decision arose from inside, a decision to *trust* in what was happening *no matter what*. It was a decision to know with certainty that it was all somehow a gift from God, and though I couldn't fully understand its mystery, I knew in time the gift would be revealed.

In that decision to trust came complete surrender. In surrender a presence of love filled the room and permeated everywhere. I was bathed in it, embraced in it. Yet I also knew it to be who *I am*. Alive, scintillating, the presence of love was *everywhere,* and there was no place I could go where it was not.

Source had been teaching me so profoundly, using my life as the classroom. With the tumor: you are not your body. With the fire: you are not your material possessions. With the IRS: you are not your money or your ability to survive. With Kelley: you are not your relationships. With Don: you are not the romance or the marriage. **You are this love that is present when all else comes and goes.**

Bodies wither and die. Possessions leave, relationships leave, lifestyles leave; but you are this love that is present when all else has come and all has gone. Eternal love. The only *real* love. The only thing that cannot come and cannot go. This was the *one* beloved worth being true to. This was the one love worth making a marriage with. I made a vow that I would be true to this beloved for the rest of my life. I would make my life an endless prayer of gratitude in surrender to this love that is here when all else had forsaken me.

I was reminded of the story "Footprints":

One night a man had a dream.

He dreamed he was walking along the beach with the Lord. Across the sky flashed scenes from his life. For each scene, he noticed two sets of footprints in the sand; one belonged to him and the other to the Lord.

When the last scene of his life flashed before him, he looked back at the footprints in the sand.

He noticed that many times along the path of his life there was only one set of footprints. He also noticed that it happened at the very lowest and saddest times in his life. This really bothered him and he questioned the Lord about it.

"Lord, you said that once I decided to follow you, you'd walk with me all the way. But I have noticed that during the most troublesome times in my life, there is only one set of footprints. I don't understand why when I needed you most you would leave me."

The Lord replied, "My precious, precious child, I love you and would never leave you. During your times of trial and suffering, when you see only one set of footprints, it was then that I carried you."

This was the first time the story really had a true meaning for me. Here, in the most devastating moments of my life, Source was here, carrying me, embracing me. *Not two, just one.*

Don came to me later, and told me what I already knew to be true—that he still loved me deeply and that he was confused. We had a long-standing emotional issue that had not yet been resolved, and which was troubling him deeply. He also confided his confusion with his romance with Karen, and pleaded that I give him time to get clear, that I honor the twenty years of the love that we had shared.

I agreed, and made a secret vow to myself that no matter what happened, no matter how painful it became, I would not do anything to stain or dump on the sacredness of the love we *had* shared. I knew that the possibility existed that he might leave, and I decided I was not going to let twenty years of a "legendary romance" be marred by the necessary grief and pain that would have to take place. I would allow grief to be grief, and twenty years of beauty to remain twenty years of beauty.

At that same time, I also made a vow to myself that I would not start calling all my friends and family and start gossiping about myself, drawing them into the drama under the guise of "needing to confide." It felt to me a sacred time, a precious time, and I didn't want to invite everyone else's judgment and projected pain to be dumped onto what was for me a time of tremendous learning, and full recognition of what *real* love was.

So, I kept it to myself, being present day by day to whatever emotions came and went in this vast ocean of love that was omnipresent. The love was there waking, sleeping, while eatment

ing—it would not leave me, nor would I leave it. And yet the whole drama of life continued in its tumultuous ways even as I bathed in its presence.

It seemed that this love was completely untouched by any emotion that came through it, or by any circumstances that took place. It was like resting in an ocean of love in which all the drama of the fishes was taking place, and yet the ocean remained untouched by it.

Don promised he would be open with me, and share with me what was really going on for him in his heart. And though it was painful to remain "open," while I watched my husband of twenty years carrying on a long-distance romance in my presence, at least there was a power of being absolutely honest with each other. Don was my best friend, and I knew he was the one I could rely on to see me through this most painful of times.

He went off on a business trip, and Karen joined him while he was there. On his first phone call, he spoke openly about his feelings—what was coming up for him. He was still uncertain as to what it all meant, or where it would take him. Oddly, I was comforted by the obvious honesty, feeling that as long as we had clear and open communication, there would be truth in what was taking place.

However, by the end of the weekend, when he called in, I could hear a covering very clearly in his voice. A veil had come down, and pure open truth was no longer there. Out of the ocean of stillness I was resting in, a huge wave of rage began to give rise to itself. It was unlike anything I had ever experienced. The power of it was almost overwhelming, and as I listened to his covered tones, everything inside of me was raging, "THIS IS NOT RIGHT!"

The rage was enormous, and yet it seemed strangely impersonal. It didn't even feel like "I" was enraged, but that Truth itself was enraged and had a life force of its own. It felt like Truth had been given a voice, and like a volcano it exploded forth without any pretense or nicety. I'm sure it was the first time in our marriage Don had ever experienced anything like it. It was certainly the first time I ever had. I got off the phone and could feel the power of the rage building, as if a volcano was ready to blast.

Still resting in Source, I sat down on my meditation cushion. The words *"This is not right"* blasted out of my mouth. I thought to myself, "I got a tumor because I wasn't able to be present and allow myself to feel what was going on. Well, this is one time I'm *not* going to stuff it back down. I'm not going to create another tumor. I'm going to just sit here and allow the rage to be *fully* felt. I'm going to be fully present to it."

Suddenly, I began to feel a pain at the base of my spine and in my groin area. As I sat, I felt the rage turn into a blazing white-hot flame that began to burn up through my body. It came up through my belly into my stomach, leaving me red and perspiring in the wake of its fire. It continued up through my chest and into my throat, and finally seemed to leave through the top of my head.

The white flame had purified my body, and I sat there sweating, blazing in Freedom and a profound stillness. Then the next wave of emotion came; a grief and loss unlike anything I'd ever experienced. Once again, I was present to it and allowed the fullness of it to be felt. I was doubled over in pain. It too was followed by a quiet, and then the next wave of pain came; anguish. I found myself curled up in a fetal position as it poured through my body. Then once again, silence. The next wave came. Every imaginable emotion burned its way through my body.

The process lasted for six days. I lost eleven pounds in weight. At the end, I was left washed clean. The grief and loss had finished itself completely and utterly in under one week. I had not known that just allowing pure raw emotion to come through the body could be that painful, but what I learned was that if you are *fully* present to it, if you welcome it, *there is no pain—no matter how deep—that cannot finish itself this quickly.* I was left in a wake of peace that is still with me today.

I've subsequently heard it said in spiritual circles, that if you are totally present to grief, all grief will finish itself in five to seven days. There is *no* grief so great that it needs to last longer than that. Grief is prolonged either because we don't let it all come up, or worse, because we string it out by believing our society's dictum that it has to last longer.

All this had taken place, and still the presence of love in which I was resting was completely untouched by it. Even in the depth of anguish, love was there. It was as if the body had to go through this profound and powerful letting-go process, even though "I" was identified with love itself. Love remained when all else left.

And so it went for the next couple of months—love present, while the drama of life continued. Finally, there came a point where I said to Don, "You must make up your mind. I'm surrendered to whatever decision is made. I just want somewhere to give my life into. If we're to remain married, please let me give my life to that, or if I'm to be single, then please let me give my life to that, but please give me some place to surrender."

He said he needed time to go into silence and truly get clear, as I was forcing him to make his decision before he was really ready. He was going to Hawaii for a seminar, and he promised that while he was there, he would be still and come to a decision.

On his way out the door, I looked into his pained eyes. It was clear that this was also the hardest thing that he had been through in his life, and quietly he said, "I know this sounds like bullshit, but underneath it all, I've had this incessant deep feeling that I'm doing this all for you. I don't know what I mean by that, but that's what's been coming up for me."

I answered that perhaps he was right, and when he closed the door something inside of me knew it was true. I didn't know how, but I *knew* it was true.

While Don was in Hawaii, I continued to rest in awareness, life still happening in a bath of love. I had noticed that ever since the "This is not right" day, I had a nagging feeling gnawing at my guts. Every morning, just as I was waking up, I could feel my tummy churn. When I finally asked myself, "What am I really feeling?," inwardly I heard the simple word *betrayal*. The grief, loss, and pain had finished completely, but the feeling of betrayal still haunted me.

So I decided it was time to call my close friend Vicki, and finally let her know everything that was taking place. I knew I needed an Emotional Journey process big time, and as I was still "hooked" with the betrayal issue, I hoped she would be willing to help me out.

When she heard the news she said, "Of course, Brandon. Come over today. Bring the Emotional Journey script with you, as I'm a bit rusty. I haven't done one in a while, and this is a pretty big issue."

As we sat there for the process, my tummy began to flutter, as it always does right before I start a Journey process. I truly didn't know what I would encounter. I had been so present to all my emotions, and I couldn't figure out why it was that this particular one wouldn't stop nagging me.

It took almost no time to go through the layers, and when we got to the campfire, Vicki said, "Well, as this is a current issue, does the seven-year-old you really need to speak to Don? The seven-year-old didn't even know Don."

"I don't know. She must be here for some reason. I suppose it can't hurt." Boy, was I surprised. It wasn't the present-day me that felt betrayed at all! It was the *younger* me that was so upset. I had made a vow to myself at seven years old that one day I would marry my "Prince Charming," and we would be madly in love and live happily ever after until the day we died. The younger me felt crushed that her storybook romance had been shattered.

A deep feeling of disillusionment and loss came as she surrendered to the truth that the romance was over. The younger me wept tears of surrender and said something totally unexpected: "It was I who betrayed myself. I believed that fairy tales can come true, and I hated you for proving me wrong, when actually, I was the one who made up the story in the first place. I was the one who took up residence and lived in the fairy tale."

When she forgave, I knew the storybook romance was finally over. I was left in the tender sweet wake of reality itself. I thought, "Isn't this amazing? Here I am, resting in this ocean of love, and still this old issue needed resolving. Thank God for the Journey process!" When I was done, I felt completely and utterly free, and have remained so ever since.

I had finally learned what it was Source had been trying to teach me—nothing you can do can give you this love. No career can give it to you; no amount of service can make you know it; no lover, partner, or family can make it happen; no house, car, or material belongings can buy it for you. Nothing and no one can give it to you, for it is who you already are. *You* are the love that you have been seeking.

It turned out Don had been right, I didn't realize that he would be the one to make my deepest, most heartfelt prayer come true. Ten years before this whole story began, I had attended a seminar with Tony Robbins, in which I uncovered my life's purpose. This purpose I memorized, inscribed on my heart, and did my best to live each day. It read, "The purpose of my life is to be pure joy, and to help myself and others discover our greatness—our god-selves."

Each day, I put out that intention, and here it was my prayer had finally been answered—it had finally come true. I had discovered what *real* joy was, and had finally uncovered what true greatness—god-self—was. Don had simply been a vehicle used in the answer to my prayer.

I had to discover for myself both what love *is* and what love is *not*, in order to uncover true greatness. What I didn't realize was that he set me free to do what it is I am here to do, for since his leave-taking I have finally been able to give my whole life into serving Truth.

So much of my energy and devotion had been focused on Don and his career. Now I was free to give all my love into serving humankind in waking up to the Freedom and love that is what we truly are. I am sitting here today, writing this book, because I was finally set free to do what had been my deepest heart's desire. I am living my soul's purpose.

Kelley finally got in touch with me a year later, and came to her first Journey seminar in London. There were many tears of joy and renewal of our deep love, and a year later I was privileged to be there with her as she gave birth to our beautiful grandchild, Claire Grace.

Since then I have been going on tour around the world, giving Journey workshops. As the Journey grew I found the need to take on a business partner. Over time, very slowly and sweetly, a soft romance crept in on cat's paws. Kevin and I were married on Maui, in January 1998.

His commitment to serving Truth is equal to my own, and together we are deeply fulfilled in the knowledge that love cannot be given or received. It's who you are. And still, it is a great joy to celebrate life together in this ocean of love.

Ultimately, life is the *real* journey.

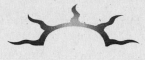

29

Tools Section

Important Note

You *must* have read this book before beginning process work. It is *essential* that you *fully understand the work,* and have heard several experiences and learned the various aspects of it *before you start your own process.*

General Instructions for Process Work

As you know, the processes can be powerfully heart opening and humbling, so it is important that you honor your own process by setting aside at least two hours of uninterrupted time in a quiet, nurturing environment. Turn off your phones and create a "sacred space" for you and your partner.

It's best to work with someone who has already read this book, who is both supportive of the work and who feels committed to serving you in your process. You both should familiarize your-selves with the process by reading it through a couple of times, just so there are no surprises in the wording or content.

Then, I recommend you begin by making a silent prayer or intention, seeing yourself and your partner as already whole; committing to be open like a child, honest and trusting of both yourself and the process. Also, make a commitment to support your partner with that same love and respect. Then sit quietly for a few moments in stillness.

Emotional Journey Instructions

To begin, first read and follow the General Instructions. You'll need to copy out the Worksheets onto a separate piece of paper and have a pen ready.

In the Emotional Journey, as you are dropping down through the layers, it is essential to **stay out of the story**—out of your analytical thoughts—and put all your attention and awareness onto **feeling the pure raw emotion** *in your body*.

Just feel the feeling fully, name it, and drop through to the next feeling. Feel it fully, rawly, intensely and drop through to the next feeling. You keep dropping through from one emotional feeling to the next, until you finally experience Source.

This is *not* a process about listening to your mind-talk and analyzing why you are feeling what you are feeling. It simply is a process of dropping through the emotional layers, like peeling back the layers of an onion, to get to the core of your being, to Source.

At the top of the sheets, the instructions advise you, whenever you see ". . ." to pause, and allow your partner "sufficient" time to experience the answer to your question. Sufficient time can be ten to fifteen seconds for some, or forty-five seconds to a minute for others.

What is important to understand is that the point of the process is to feel the emotions strongly and, after tasting each one fully, immediately drop through to the next layer. It is not necessary, nor is it a good idea, to wallow in the emotion at every level. Nor is it advisable to describe it in detail and tell a story about it.

To access feelings, rather than consult your thoughts, just internally scan your body and find where the emotion feels strongest. It may start as a subtle sensation. As you focus your attention on it, ask for it to intensify itself. Be willing to experience the power of it. Keep your attention on the feeling inside your body.

Then, very simply, feel it and drop through; feel it and drop through.

At some point you may feel yourself devoid of feeling. You might describe it as a numbness or a confusion, or an "I don't knowness," or a black hole or a void, or a nothingness, or even a feeling of being "stuck."

This is part of the process. *Everyone* **goes through this "unknown" layer. I call it the "unknown zone." It is the gateway to Source.**

When your partner names any one of these words, know that it is just another feeling layer. Encourage them to experience it fully, *relax* and drop through.

If you find they are struggling at all with the black hole, void, nothingness, then turn to the Troubleshooting pages. They will give you helpful instructions on how to help someone who feels afraid of or resistant to the "unknown zone." They will help you gracefully drop through. As your partner will have read this book, they will recognize where they are when you remind them.

It's natural to fear the unknown, so be sure to reassure your partner that they are doing fine, to relax into it, surrender and drop through.

After they have dropped through the unknown zone, usually your partner will start feeling lighter and easier, and a great sense of relief will gradually start taking place.

It's important to continue taking them down through the remaining levels until they reach Source. You'll know they are in Source when they experience themselves as *very vast*—as a presence that is both inside and outside the body—*everywhere.*

This is a very important point to understand, because often after dropping through the unknown zone, your partner will start using Sourcelike words such as love, peace, laughter, joy, light, contentment, freedom, *but* they may still feel it's located somewhere *inside* the body.

It's when the feeling becomes very expansive, spacious—as if they are one with everything, or are part of everything—that it is a true realization of Source. When it is vast, it moves from being a simple emotion to being pure awareness itself.

Once your partner feels this vast spaciousness, you can let them rest there for about thirty seconds. Then follow the script, bringing Source up through each level in turn.

You'll find your asterisk (*) marking where people first showed up. That will be your Campfire Level. If no people show up going down through the levels, then choose the strongest emotion which appeared before the unknown zone (excluding the starting level). You can begin your Campfire Process there.

Once you are at the campfire, make certain that your partner is saying what *really* needs to be said. The campfire is there so that the younger you can empty yourself completely of all the emotions that were felt, but usually not expressed, at the time. So make certain that everything that *needs* to be said gets spoken out loud. It is essential that the younger you gets everything off their chest.

Once your partner feels empty and complete, then you can ask if they are ready to forgive. In order to forgive *authentically*, a person really needs to be empty.

If, for any reason, they feel they are not ready to forgive, then ask the mentor, **"What would have to happen in order to forgive?"** Usually, the mentor, being a higher wisdom, will give the answer that is appropriate for that person. Most often, it's just that the younger you hasn't got everything off their chest, and needs to say a few more things.

The mentor is there to assist with *any* queries that might come up. Your partner's own wisdom *knows* exactly what needs to take place. **So, when in doubt, ask the mentor**.

When the campfire is complete, you go through the Future Integration with your partner. You don't need to write it all down. It's enough just to read it. It's your way of checking with your partner that the healing will continue to evolve over time.

By six months to a year, at longest, they should be feeling lighter or easier about the emotional issue they started with. It's not necessary that they actually "see" into the future, but rather, that they can just sense or feel it.

If for any reason it appears that they are feeling no change, it's usually an indication that something wasn't completed at the campfire. This is no problem. Simply take them directly back to the campfire, and ask the mentor what else needs to be said in order to complete. Generally speaking, when forgiveness is "completely complete," the issue will leave. When done with the campfire, go back through the Future Integration freshly.

When it's all done, hand to your partner a sheet of paper and a pen, and let them write their Letter to Themselves in their own time. You might like to get them a glass of water, or a cup of tea, and suggest they keep the letter somewhere visible, where they can read it each day.

Then, if you'd like, it's time for you to switch.

When you're both done, it's good to take some time to let the work integrate. Have a hot bath, some hot soup, and a nap or rest.

Sometimes, after finishing a process, you can feel a little tender or vulnerable, or even a little disoriented for a short while—as the healing is beginning to take place inside the body. It's important to realize that this is a *positive signal* that healing is taking place.

If you do feel disoriented or a little woozy, it's best not to drive or do anything strenuous or requiring concentration. Give yourself some time to come around fully.

Very often it can happen that, over the next few days, flashbacks of related memories may come floating through consciousness, or even strong emotions may seem to arise out of nowhere. This is wonderful! Know that this is just the residual emotional toxicity continuing to move out, and let it wash through you. It's a sign that the healing is continuing. If strong emotions come, just let them come up, and they will wash up and wash out. Treat them in the same way you would if physical toxicity were to happen. If you found yourself vomiting up something toxic that you had eaten, you wouldn't then pull it apart, analyze it, and try to stuff it back down—would you?

In the same way, if old emotions come washing up, just don't touch them. Just let them come and let them go. I always suggest at the seminars that you just **"Stop, breathe and be present"** to any emotion—and it will wash up and wash through.

Be honoring of yourself and your process, and let your body heal in its time. Trust yourself and the process. It has already helped thousands to free themselves from long-standing emotional challenges.

Important Note

There is no way it can hurt you or your partner to go down through the emotional layers. The worst (or best) that can happen is that your partner actually feels the strong emotions already stored inside their body. Even if you were to stop in midstream, all that would happen is that your partner would open their eyes having experienced some strong emotions—that's all!

All *pure* emotions simply come and simply go. The only thing that makes an emotion *stay* is telling yourself a story about it, or wasting time analyzing it, or listening to mind-talk about it.

No emotion can last more than a few moments if you are truly authentic. Have you ever noticed with babies? One moment they are crying, then someone shakes a rattle and the next moment they are laughing and gurgling. They don't feel the need to hold on to the previous emotion, in order to be consistent. They don't need to prove to themselves how important or significant the emotion is. They just feel it and move on to the next moment.

So, know that you are perfectly safe going down through the levels—no matter what the emotion, no matter how strong. If you are really real it will come and it will go.

Some people say, "I'm afraid of opening a can of worms." The only can of worms you can open is listening to your mind-talk selling you a story about your emotions. Emotions, in and of themselves, are healthy. Being able to feel is a wholesome and natural part of being human. What is not natural is listening to your mind analyze, blame, and make up stories about the emotions.

So know that feeling emotions is healthy. With any emotion, just stop, breathe, and be present. It will come and it will go.

Physical Journey Instructions

Begin by reading the General Instructions as well as the Emotional Journey instructions. Then read through the Physical Journey sheets a few times to refamiliarize yourself with the process.

It is preferable to use the Physical Journey only *after* someone has already been through the Emotional Journey, because it makes the assumption that your partner has already had a direct personal experience of Source.

The Physical Journey can flow very easily, and can be read almost like a fairy tale or a guided meditation. Remember to take your time and be gentle as you read this process. Pause whenever you see "...".

You might like to softly emphasize any words that are capitalized, and it can be very helpful to breathe at the same pace that your partner is breathing. It's best to speak in soft tones as you guide them through the process.

Some people don't visualize well. That's absolutely fine. It's enough to get a sense or a knowing about what it's like inside. Some people may actually see accurate anatomical pictures, while others may come up with more metaphorical images. Some may not see anything at all, and will just feel the texture, or sense or know what it's like inside. Others may hear words describing what it's like. Everyone is unique, so let your partner have their own unique discovery.

When you get to the Change Memory Process, you'll notice that you'll be asking your partner to come up with some "resource balloons." Often, when your partner is immersed in the process, they may feel so "deep" that they cannot immediately come up with any emotional resources. It's kind to offer them suggestions at this point. Use your common sense, and trust that you will be able to make some useful suggestions. There are some emotional resources that I almost always use: self-worth, creativity in communication, wisdom, Source, light-heartedness, sense of humor, the ability to get through, the ability to take appropriate action, the ability to ask for help, self-love, self-confidence, and a crystal dome that allows others' negative emotions to roll off. You may find some of these resources useful in your own process.

The Campfire Process is similar to the Emotional Journey campfire, so please read those instructions carefully before starting this process.

When you are complete, make sure you give your partner plenty of time to watch the transformation inside the body. It can be quite an extraordinary and wondrous experience.

Lastly, trust yourself and trust the process. It is a wonderful adventure.

Instructions for Children's Work

Begin by reading *all* of the previous instructions.

When working with children up to the age of fourteen, I strongly suggest using the Physical Journey *only*. For most children, it will read like a fairy tale, and will feel playful and fun to do.

Before you begin, you might like to discuss with your child various inner qualities that heroes have—qualities like love, compassion, inner strength, sense of humor, ability to express themselves, honesty. In this way your child will be aware of possible inner resourceful states before the process begins.

In working with children, it is important to be aware that they have very quick access to their imaginations and creative abilities, and they may race ahead of your pace in the process. They may run down the staircase, jump into the space shuttle, and end up somewhere inside the body before you've even finished your words. So, please make sure you keep up with them!

In children's work, we always ask a hero to appear, rather than a mentor, as all children know what a hero is and they trust the hero's strength and wisdom.

Children will likely have very vivid pictures of what it's like inside the body. It's delightful to give them time to describe it in detail.

In the Change Memory Process, please feel free to suggest some inner resources that might be useful to put in the balloons. Also, your child will remember the qualities of a hero that you discussed before the process, so they might like to choose some of these as well.

When it comes to forgiveness, many young children don't yet know what the word means, so you can encourage them to say, "I'm sorry—it's okay," and then add, "I forgive you," if they understand its meaning.

When the campfire is over, give the child extra time to see how things are changing and transforming in the body. They love this part, and can be very descriptive.

Usually, when this is over, they feel impatient to get into the space shuttle and right back to the door, and often they *run* back up the stairs. Once again, let them go at their own pace.

Most children's Physical Journeys last only eleven to eighteen minutes, as children are quick to catch onto the process, find it easy to forgive, are quick to let go of the old issues, and are eager to finish. Please be sensitive to the pace your child wants to go at.

Trust your child and trust the process. Children usually love it, and often enjoy painting before-and-after pictures of how they felt.

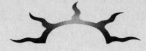

30

Process Sheets

The Emotional Journey—Overview

◈ Remember to TAKE YOUR TIME—give your partner a chance to fully identify and experience their feeling before moving on.

◈ TRUST that whatever your partner says is PERFECT.

◈ Most of all TRUST YOURSELF AND THE PROCESS.

> The object is to drop through our levels to the Source of our Being, and then bring that Source back up through the levels and illumine them.

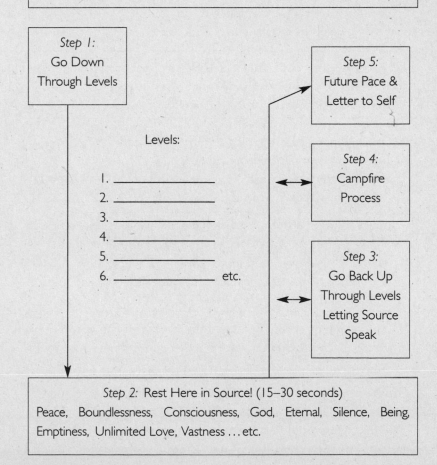

Step 1: Go Down Through Levels

Step 5: Future Pace & Letter to Self

Step 4: Campfire Process

Step 3: Go Back Up Through Levels Letting Source Speak

Levels:

1. _____
2. _____
3. _____
4. _____
5. _____
6. _____ etc.

Step 2: Rest Here in Source! (15–30 seconds)
Peace, Boundlessness, Consciousness, God, Eternal, Silence, Being, Emptiness, Unlimited Love, Vastness ... etc.

The Emotional Journey Process

> Read slowly and carefully. Whenever you see ". . ." pause and give your partner sufficient time to fully experience the pure, raw emotion.

Start by asking what your partner's emotional issue is. Write on separate worksheets that you have prepared to match the one in the book (p.179).

1. **Say:**
   "Feel the feeling fully . . ."
   "Where in your body do you feel it? . . ."
   "Breathe into it . . . experience it fully . . .
   allow yourself to intensify it . . ."

> Make sure they have time to FULLY experience the feeling, but don't let them wallow—once they have fully experienced, MOVE ON.

   "Staying open, ask yourself . . . What is beneath it? . . ."
   "Just allow yourself to drop through . . ."
   "So, what are you feeling? . . . (it may not be what you expect)"
   —Make sure they NAME the new feeling—

> At EVERY LEVEL ask, "Are there any specific people related to this feeling?" Put an asterisk at the level that the person(s) appeared, and note who was there. Once they have named a person, *stop asking this question*—you have now established the level of the CAMPFIRE.

2. Keep dropping through to the next level until you get to their Source. Let your partner rest there for approximately 15 to 30 seconds.

> Source may be called one of many names but will be boundaryless, and will have a vast quality such as: Freedom, Silence, Unlimited Peace, Eternal, Eternity, God, Unlimited Love, Consciousness, Awareness, Emptiness, Vastness.

3. **Then say:** "Knowing yourself as this vast boundlessness, this stillness, this pure love, this _____ *(person's Source)*, if _____ *(Source)* had something to say to _____ *(last level)*, what would it say?"

Wait until they answer . . .

Then say: "Just allow _____ *(Source)* to wash right through _____ *(last level)*."

4. Repeat question 3, bringing their Source up through each level until you reach the Campfire level *(the level at which you marked an asterisk)*.

5. Begin the Campfire Process *(see Campfire Process Sheet below)*. When complete, continue to point no. 6.

6. *After* completing the Campfire Process, continue bringing their Source up through the final levels repeating question 3 and washing through, until you reach their original starting level.

7. Read Future Integration, at moderate pace. There is no need to write anything down *(see Integration Process Sheet, p.176)*.

8. Give your partner a pen and paper for their letter to themselves. Let them take as much time as they need to write. You should continue sending SILENT blessings as your partner is writing.

9. With great respect and love, acknowledge each other for experiencing this process. You may wish to get some water. Stay in the energy, and switch.

The Emotional Journey—Campfire

Read slowly and carefully. Whenever you see ". . ." pause and give your partner sufficient time to fully experience the answer to your questions.

Imagine a campfire . . . the nature of which is eternal silence, unconditional love. Imagine a **younger you** sitting at this fire . . .

Now picture the **present you** sitting at the fire . . . Also at this fire is a **mentor** whose divine wisdom you trust—it can be someone you know or would like to know, a saint, a sage, or someone born of your imagination—someone in whose presence you feel safe . . . Now bring to the fire the specific people who are involved with your issue . . . who else needs to be at this campfire? . . . *(let answer)*.

Can you see the campfire? . . . Can you see the **younger you**? . . . The **present you**? . . . The **mentor**? . . . Who else is there? . . . *(let them answer—write down the names so you can refer to them specifically, i.e., Mother, Father, Loved One, etc.)* Of the people involved with your issue, ask the **younger you** to which ONE or TWO would you like to speak? . . . *(If two people, ask: To whom would you like to speak first?)*

Go through **all** questions (1 to 11) for **each** person spoken to.

1. Everyone is now sitting in the protective presence of this fire of unconditional love and acceptance. The **younger you** may have experienced a great deal of pain in the past. Let the **younger you** speak now from that previous pain, saying what needs to be said, and letting _____ *(Mother, Father, Loved One, etc.)* hear what needs to be heard . . . *(long pause)*.

2. Knowing that _____ *(Mother, Father, Loved One, etc.)* was probably doing the best he/she could with the resources he/she had at the time, let him/her reply . . . *(pause for reply)*.

3. What does the **younger you** have to reply to that? . . . *(let answer)*.

4. If _____ *(Mother, Father, Loved One, etc.)* were to reply, not from the level of the personality, but from the level of the soul, what might he/she say? . . . *(let answer)*.

5. How does the **younger you** reply to that? . . . *(continue until empty)*.

6. Does the **mentor** have anything to add? . . . *(let answer)*.

7. What does the **present you** have to say to _____ *(Mother, Father, Loved One, etc.)*? . . . *(continue until empty)*.

8. What would _____ *(Mother, Father, Loved One, etc.)* reply from the level of the soul? . . . *(let answer)*.

9. Does anyone have anything more to add? . . . *(continue conversation until empty)*.

10. When the **younger you** is ready, ask: "Even though his/her previous behavior may not have been acceptable by **any** standards, and even if you in no way condone his/her behavior, are you willing to **completely and utterly** forgive him/her from the bottom of your heart?" . . . *(let answer)*. Now go ahead and forgive him/her . . . *(let forgive)*.

11. When the **present you** is ready, ask: "Even though his/her previous behavior may not have been acceptable by **any** standards, and even if you in no way condone his/her behavior, are you willing to **completely and utterly** forgive him/her from the bottom of your heart?" . . . *(wait for answer)*. Now go ahead and forgive him/her . . . *(let forgive)*.

> Now repeat process of questions 1 to 11 for the **second person** to be addressed, so that all is said and heard. When this is completed, continue by saying the following:

Say: Go ahead and forgive them all, sending them blessings. Allow them to merge into the fire, which is the source of all life . . . Then turn to the **younger you** and say: "I promise you will **never** have to experience this previous pain again. I forgive you for any pain which was caused, because you just didn't have access to the resources that I do now, and I promise you can have access to them any time you like. I love you and will always protect you." . . . Then, hugging the **younger you**, let yourself merge, allowing the **younger you** to grow up with this forgiveness inside . . . Turning to the **mentor**, thank him/her . . . Now come back to the present and we will continue going up through the remaining levels.

At **each** remaining level **ask:** "Knowing yourself as this vast boundlessness, this stillness, this pure love, this _____ *(person's*

Source), if _____ (Source) had something to say to _____
(last level), what would it say? . . ."

Wait for answer . . .

Then say: "Just allow _____ *(Source)* to wash over _____
(last level)."

> When all levels are completed go on to Future Integration
> (below).

The Emotional Journey—Integration Process

> Read at a moderate pace. Whenever you see ". . ." give a short
> pause and allow your partner to experience the process. You
> needn't write anything down.

"Having learned what you've learned, having experienced what
you've experienced—see yourself a day from now . . . What do
you feel like? . . . What kind of things are you doing? . . .
Saying? . . . Feeling? . . . How do you feel about yourself? . . .

"Now see yourself a week from now. What do you look like? . . .
What kinds of things are you saying to yourself? . . . What kinds
of actions are you taking? . . . What are you feeling? . . .

"Now picture yourself a month from now—how are you feeling
in your body? . . . Are you feeling free, confident, and light? . . .
What are you saying to yourself? . . . What are you doing? . . .
How does your body feel? . . . What if that old issue tried to give
rise to itself? . . . What does _____ *(Source)* say to it? . . . How
are you handling it? . . .

"Now see yourself six months down the line—how are you feeling? . . . about yourself? . . . about life? . . . Do you know at this

point that already 70 percent of your cells are all new? . . . You are literally becoming all new . . . What if that old issue tried to give rise to itself ? . . . How are you handling it now? . . .

"Now picture yourself one year from now—what do you look like? . . . How are you feeling about yourself? . . . Are you aware that not a single molecule that was here a year ago is here today—you are literally all new? . . . Can you even imagine that old issue trying to give rise to itself ? . . . Is it even possible for it to do so? . . . What does _____ *(Source)* say? . . . Is handling this old issue a breeze? . . .

"Now picture yourself five years from now—how are you feeling? . . . Does this old behavior even come up anymore? . . . How does your body feel? . . . How do you feel about life? . . .

"Now see yourself ten years down the road—are you feeling so free from this old pattern that it doesn't seem possible or real? . . . How are you handling things? . . . How do you feel about yourself and your life? . . .

"Now, staying connected to the *future you—to the Source of you ten years from now*—what advice would you give to the present you? . . . What beliefs would help you most now? . . . What actions would serve you most now? . . . What are some daily things you could do and say to yourself? . . .

"With soft eyes—open your eyes slowly, *staying connected to the future you*. Let the future you write a letter to the present you, giving practical advice on how to be . . . what to believe . . . what kind of action to take . . . what kind of physiology is useful . . . what to say to yourself . . . what to say to others . . . what you can do on a daily basis . . . *Let the free, wise future you guide you now!* You may open your eyes now when you are ready."

The Emotional Journey—Letter to Yourself

With soft eyes—open your eyes slowly, staying connected to the future you. Let the future you write a letter to the present you, giving practical advice on how to be . . . what to believe . . . what you have learned that will continue to unfold and benefit you from now on . . . what kinds of actions to take . . . what kind of physiology is useful . . . what to say to yourself . . . what to say to others . . . what you can do on a daily basis . . .

Let the free, wise future you guide you now!

My Dear Self,

The Emotional Journey Worksheet

Worksheet For: (Name)	

Emotion	Where in Body	What Source says to each level on way back up
→		←
→		←
→		←
→		←
→		←
→		←
→		←
→		←

At every level ask "Are there any specific people related to this feeling?"
As soon as someone appears, mark an asterisk (*) at that level and STOP ASKING THIS QUESTION. You have now established the Campfire Level

SOURCE:_____

The Emotional Journey—Troubleshooting

1. BEING STUCK

> *If your partner says they are stuck (or "don't know"), know that stuck (or not knowing) is just another level.*

Say:
GREAT! This is a pattern you've run before. You've been here before in your life . . .
Feel the feeling of being stuck (or not knowing) completely . . .
Breathe into being stuck (or not knowing) . . .
Where in your body do you feel this stuck feeling (or not knowing)? . . .
On a scale of 1 to 10, make it 100!
I wonder what would happen if you were to smile and relax at being stuck (or not knowing) . . . This is the gateway to who you really are . . .
What is beneath it? . . .
Stay open and curious like a child—it may not be quite what you'd expect . . .
Just allow yourself to drop through/be guided through . . .

2. BLACK HOLE/VOID

> *Congratulate and Celebrate! Always reassure, never make wrong!*

Say:
GREAT! You've spent your whole life avoiding this place!
I wonder what would happen if you were to smile and relax into the Black Hole/Void? . . .
This is the place you've avoided all your life—now you have the courage to face it . . .
I wonder what it is that's shining right behind the darkness—what's coming through the cracks or pinholes? . . . What's seeping into the darkness? . . .
Pay very close attention to what is shining there . . .

Stay open and curious like a child—it may not be quite what you'd expect . . .
Then after a few seconds, say:
What's happening in your body right now? . . .
This feeling may be quiet as a whisper. . . .
What is *that* feeling? . . .

3. TROUBLE FEELING THE EMOTIONS

If your partner is having TROUBLE FEELING THEIR EMOTIONS and is TALKING TOO MUCH, have them STOP their story—they are in their head, not their body. Have them tune in to and focus on what they are feeling in their body.

Say:
Intensify the feeling in your body . . .
Feel it fully—where in your body do you feel it? . . .
Breathe into the feeling . . .
This feeling may be as quiet as a whisper . . .
What is happening in your body right now? . . . Pay close attention—it may be very subtle . . .
What is that feeling? . . .

MOST IMPORTANT: TRUST YOURSELF AND TRUST THE PROCESS. *RELAX, SMILE, AND ENJOY!*

The Ten Steps to the Physical Journey

> Read slowly and carefully. Whenever you see ". . ." pause and give your partner *sufficient time* to fully experience and answer your questions.

1. **Guide** your partner into **Source**.
2. Take **Shuttle Ride** with mentor on **Journey of Discovery**.
3. Walk around and **explore** the region.
4. **Uncover emotion** and associated **memory** or people.
5. Guide partner through **Memory Process**.
6. Guide partner through **Campfire Process**.
7. **See** how region has **changed**.
8. Take **Shuttle** back to:
   a) doorway where we started (for all workshop processes).
   b) different part of body (not for workshop processes).
9. If Journeying to a different part of the body, repeat steps 2–8.
10. **Guide** partner back to **waking consciousness**.

> Thank your partner and share your experiences of the process. Get up, walk around a little, get a glass of water—then switch.

The Physical Journey—Going to Source

> Read slowly and carefully. Whenever you see ". . ." pause and give your partner *sufficient time* to fully experience and answer your questions.

Allow yourself to find a comfortable position, and when you're ready, you may close your eyes. . . . As you feel yourself sitting in your chair . . . and as you hear the sounds in the room . . . and as you feel your breath gently going in and going out, you may begin to feel yourself RELAX. . . . And as you hear the sound of my voice, and as you feel your back resting against the chair . . . and with every breath you take, you may begin to notice that it is CAUSING you to RELAX . . . deeper and deeper . . . more and more relaxed . . . into your very Source.

Imagine a downward-facing staircase in front of you . . . there are 10 steps . . . Can you see it? . . . or get a sense of it? . . . *(give time to answer)* . . . Good . . . Now in your mind's eye, go ahead and step onto step number 10, the top step . . . Now step onto the next step—step 9 . . . now 8 . . . With each step you take it is drawing you deeper and deeper into your Source . . . Now step onto step 7 . . . 6 . . . 5 . . . Just allow yourself to relax deeper into yourself with every step you take . . . 4 . . . 3 . . . expanding and allowing yourself to go deeper and deeper . . . 2 . . . and now, as you get ready to step onto the bottom step, step 1, allow yourself to extend your awareness in front of you . . . Now feel your boundlessness expand behind you . . . Now allow your awareness to extend infinitely to either side of you . . . Let space extend underneath you . . . and allow your awareness to expand above . . . Just rest in the experience of ever-deepening boundlessness . . . letting your Self grow still and silent in the ever-deepening expanse . . . 1 . . . Rest in the awareness of your Self as Source . . . *(let your partner rest here for approximately 15 to 30 seconds).*

The Physical Journey—The Shuttle Ride

Now, imagine a thermometer in the ground. It has numbers going from 1 to 10. One is the deepest you can go, and 10 is refreshed, alive waking consciousness. If you can't exactly see the thermometer, that is perfectly fine . . . Can you get a sense that it is there? . . . *(give time to answer)* . . . Just know that it is there . . . Now if 1 is the deepest you can go into the Source, and 10 is full, bright waking consciousness, can you get a sense of where you are on the thermometer? . . . You may actually hear a number, or see it rise to a certain level, or just get a sense or a knowing about where you are . . . So where are you on the thermometer? . . . *(give time to answer)* . . . Can you let the thermometer rise by a half point? . . . *(give time to answer)* . . . Can you let it fall by 1 point? . . . *(give time to answer)* . . . Good . . . Now that you know exactly who's in charge, what number would you like it to be at? . . . You can just allow that to happen naturally of its own accord as you continue to let boundlessness expand in all directions, knowing it will do so perfectly of its own accord. . . .

Now imagine a door in front of you . . . behind the door is pure light . . . the light of your Being—your own Source . . . the nature of this light is boundless love . . . Also behind this door is your sage or mentor—one whose wisdom you trust, and in whose presence you feel safe and protected . . . When you are ready, you may step through the door into your own light and greet your mentor . . . *(give time)* . . . Have you stepped through? . . . Good . . . Have you greeted your mentor? . . . Good.

Now imagine a space shuttle in front of you . . . This space shuttle is a very special vehicle . . . It can take you to any part of your body, no matter how small or large, and it knows exactly where to go . . . It can go inside your organs, in your veins, muscles, or tissue in a very graceful, safe, and protected way . . . Now go ahead and let you and your mentor step inside . . . Are you inside? . . . Good . . . Now, when you are ready push the green button and let it take you to your first stop—it may not be where you expect to go—so just allow the shuttle to be your guide. It is powered by your own body wisdom . . . so let your wisdom take you where it wants to go, and when you arrive, be sure to pull on your hand brake and let me know . . . *(wait)* . . .

GO TO DISCOVERY SHEET, p. 185

The Physical Journey—Discovery Process

So, do you have a sense where you are yet? . . . *(let answer—they may not know yet, this is fine)* . . . Great . . . Go ahead and step outside the shuttle with your mentor with big flashlights in your hands . . . What does it look like? . . . What does it feel like under your feet? . . . Can you describe what the area is like? . . . Do you get the sense that you are inside or outside the organ? . . . *[if outside read the following—"imagine a small doorway somewhere, and let you and your mentor step directly into the core of this organ (or muscle or tissue)"]* . . . Now put your flashlights on high beam . . . What does it look like? . . . Are there any irregularities that sort of stand out to you, or look different from the rest of the area? . . . Take your time . . . keep walking around and really take a close look at what it's like in there . . . you don't have to *see* it exactly . . . Just get a sense of it, or an inner knowing . . . *(long pause)* . . . Is there an area or region that seems to draw your attention to it? . . . What does it look like? . . . Go right over and stand next to it . . . How does it make you feel? . . . If it had an emotional feeling radiating from it, what feeling would you say that is? . . . *(let answer)* . . . If it gave you a sense of how it feels and you had to name that feeling, what would that feeling be? . . . Allow yourself to experience the feeling fully . . . *(let them name the feeling)* . . . Breathe into it . . .

Ask yourself, "When have I felt like this before?," and in answer to this question, in your mind's eye, look down at your feet and see what, if any, shoes you are wearing . . . Look at your legs and your clothes . . . Get a sense of how old you feel yourself to be, and where you might be . . . Who else is there? . . . Does the person or people call to mind a certain memory or a series of memories? . . . *(give time to answer)* . . . Great . . .

> When a specific memory or series of memories comes to mind, go to the Memory Process Sheet (p. 186).

> If no particular memory comes to mind, repeat last paragraph. If still no memory arises go directly to Campfire Sheet (p.187), and invite the people directly related to this feeling to the campfire. Then proceed normally.

The Physical Journey—Memory Process

Now that you have uncovered a memory or series of memories . . . go ahead and put the whole scene onto a big movie screen, but for now let the screen go blank, knowing that you can have access to this memory in a moment . . . Is it on the movie screen? . . . Good . . . Have you let it go blank? . . . Great.

Now imagine that you and your mentor are sitting by a campfire right here—right where you are in this organ. The nature of this campfire is unconditional love and peace—Source itself . . . You and your mentor are filled with the love and peace of your own Source as you sit here by this fire getting ready to view the scene or series of scenes being played upon the movie screen . . . When you are ready, go ahead and play the scene, and when it's over, let the screen go blank and let me know . . . *(give lots of time)* . . . Would you be willing to describe to me what took place in the scene? . . . *(give time to answer)* . . . Now have the younger you that went through the scene step down off the screen and come over to the campfire and sit with the present you and the mentor.

Now, as you all sit peacefully at this fire, ask the present you or your mentor what kinds of resourceful states you WOULD have found useful in the scene . . . *(give time to think and come up with resourceful states—be encouraging)* . . . *(let them name them, and write down)* . . .

Now go ahead and give the younger you in the scene a bouquet of balloons containing all these resourceful states or emotions, and then put the scene up on the movie screen and see HOW IT

WOULD HAVE HAPPENED if you'd had access to all these resourceful states . . . When it's over let the screen go blank and let me know . . . *(allow sufficient time)* . . . How did it play itself out? . . . Would you give me a brief description? . . . Good.

Now I would like to ask the younger you and the other person(s) in the scene to step down off the screen. The younger you probably has some things that need to be said which were not said at that time, and the other people in the memory have some things they need to hear.

The Physical Journey—Campfire Process

Read slowly and carefully. Whenever you see ". . ." pause and give your partner *sufficient time* to fully experience and answer your questions.

Imagine a campfire . . . you can set it up right here inside the organ or tissue . . . The nature of this campfire is eternal silence, unconditional love. You and your mentor are present at this fire . . . Now bring to the fire the specific people who are involved with your issue . . . Do any other people need to be at this campfire? . . . *(let answer)*.

Can you see the campfire? . . . Can you see the younger you? . . . the present you? . . . the mentor? . . . Who else is there? . . . *(let answer, and write down all the names so you can refer to them specifically)*.

Of the people involved with your issue, to which ONE or TWO would you like to speak? . . . in the knowledge that anyone else there will hear what needs to be heard . . . To whom would you like to speak first? . . . *(let answer)*.

> Go through ALL questions (1 to 11) for EACH person to be spoken to.

1. Everyone is now sitting in the protective presence of this fire of unconditional love and acceptance. The **younger you** may have experienced a great deal of pain in the past. Let the **younger you** speak now from that previous pain, saying what needs to be said, and let _____ *(Mother, Father, Loved One, etc.)* hear what needs to be heard . . . *(long pause)*.

2. Knowing that _____ *(Mother, Father, Loved One, etc.)* was probably doing the best he/she could with the resources he/she had at the time, let him/her reply . . . *(long pause)*.

3. What does the **younger you** have to reply? . . . *(let answer)*.

4. If _____ *(Mother, Father, Loved One, etc.)* was to reply, not from the level of the personality, but from the level of the soul, what might he/she say? . . . *(let answer)*.

5. Does the **younger you** have anything to reply to that? . . . *(let answer)*.

6. Does the **mentor** have anything to add? . . . *(let answer)*.

7. What does the **present you** have to say to _____ *(Mother, Father, Loved One, etc.)?* . . . *(let answer)*.

8. What would _____ *(Mother, Father, Loved One, etc.)* reply from the level of the soul? . . . *(let answer)*.

9. Does anyone have anything more to add? . . . *(continue until empty)*.

10. When the **younger you** is ready ask: "Even though his/her previous behavior may not have been acceptable by **any** standards—even if you in no way condone his/her behavior, are you willing to **completely and utterly** forgive him/her from the bottom of your heart?" . . . *(let answer)*. Now go ahead and forgive him/her . . . *(let forgive)*.

11. When the **present you** is ready ask: "Even though his/her previous behavior may not have been acceptable by **any** standards—even if you in no way condone his/her behavior, are

you willing to **completely and utterly** forgive him/her from the bottom of your heart?" . . . *(let answer).* Now go ahead and forgive him/her . . . *(let forgive).*

> If two people are to be spoken to—repeat process of questions 1 to 11 for the second person to be addressed, so that all is said and heard. When this is completed, continue by saying the following:

Say: Go ahead and forgive them all, sending them blessings. Allow them to merge into the fire which is the source of all life . . . Then turn to the younger you and say: "I forgive you for any previous pain which was caused—you just didn't have access to the resources that I do now, and now you can have access to them any time you like. I promise you will never have to experience this again, because I love you and will always protect you." . . . Then, hugging the younger you, let yourself merge, allowing the younger you to grow up with this forgiveness and these resources inside.

Now, let the campfire disappear . . . Only you and your mentor are left . . . take out your high-beam flashlights and shine them all around . . . What do you see? . . . How are things changing? . . . *(let answer)* . . . Great . . . Is there any final communication the organ or tissue itself wants to make? . . . *(give time)* . . .

Knowing that it will continue to heal perfectly automatically of its own accord and that the part of you responsible for making your heart beat and your eyes shine and your cells replicate will continue the healing process perfectly without you even thinking about it—the way it does all the time, quite naturally while you are sleeping—you and your mentor can leave with grateful hearts.

GO TO FINAL JOURNEY HOME SHEET, p. 190

The Physical Journey—Final Journey Home to Waking Consciousness

Having completed your healing journey for today, get back into your space shuttle and let it take you and your mentor back to the doorway you first came through. Now step outside the shuttle and thank your mentor with all your heart, knowing you can go on this inner journey any time you like . . . Now walk through the doorway . . . there you will find the thermometer in the ground . . . Can you get a sense of what number you are at? . . . that's perfect . . .

Now step onto step 1 . . . and as we count back from 1 to 10 you will feel yourself becoming more refreshed, alive, and joyous . . . 2 . . . 3 . . . 4 . . . you can stretch and let your body feel more energized . . . 5 . . . 6 . . . 7 . . . becoming relaxed, refreshed, ready to wake up to full waking consciousness—grateful to yourself for taking your inner physical journey . . . 8 . . . feeling alive . . . 9 . . . and you may open your eyes ONLY as soon as all parts of you are fully integrated and ready to continue the healing process naturally on its own . . . 10 . . . you may open your eyes.

Take a moment or two to take some deep breaths. You may want to move about, get some water, stretch and then share with your partner your joint experiences.

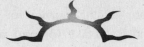

Afterword

So many people come to The Journey with physical challenges such as chronic fatigue, M.E., tumors, cancer, arthritis, chronic back pain, or acute knee pain. They may have trouble sleeping or have been diagnosed with chronic depression or are perhaps feeling listless or lethargic. Still others come with emotional issues, like debilitating rage, or they know that they are sensitive to criticism or have low self-esteem. Some come because they fear public speaking or have problems with procrastination or anxiety or stress. Still others may have challenges with smoking, drinking, or drug problems. Many come because they feel they cannot resolve the grief or loss in their life, or perhaps they have a sexual block which is holding them back from intimacy.

A great many people come because they know they are capable of achieving great things, and yet something holds them back—some "hidden comfort zone" seems to stop them from achieving the kind of abundance and success they just know they are capable of.

In each of these cases, people have succeeded in getting to the very core of their issue, be it emotional or physical, and they have been successful in setting themselves free. They have participated in their own healing process.

And yet what they go home with is something much deeper and more priceless than healing. They go home with the knowledge of who they *really* are. They come to realize that all of these emotional and physical challenges have actually turned out to be the greatest gifts of their lives because they served as a wake-up call. And what they wake up to is the immense beauty of their own soul. They wake up to the presence of love that had always been secretly tucked away in their hearts. They come for healing and they leave with the realization, the knowledge, that the kingdom of God most certainly dwells within.

With all my heart I pray that this book has given *you* a wake-up call. I hope that all the inspiring stories of self-discovery will ignite a flame of longing in your own heart and cause you to go on your own spiritual journey.

Perhaps someday I might have the joy of meeting you, or maybe you will feel inspired to pass this book along to a friend, so that each human heart can become aware of its own greatness.

May you discover the presence of love, which is your own true self, and live as a true expression of Freedom.

In all love, Brandon.

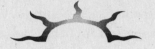

Author's Note

This book is written to inspire you to recognize and realize the greatness that lies within all of us—to point to the possibility that participating in our own healing journeys is a gift we can give to ourselves. It is a wake-up call to the freedom and wholeness already inside.

It is NOT designed to take you away from whatever healing or health program you are on—whether orthodox or alternative. Instead, it is meant to *enhance* and support your own chosen process and growth. You should feel free to use this work gracefully alongside whatever healing path you are on.

In the field of healing there are no guarantees, and there are as many routes to healing and health as there are people. Hopefully, the words in this book will inspire and support you in whatever path you choose.

If your heart feels called to know more about this work or tapes or Journey workshops, please feel free to call The Journey in the U.S.A. toll free on 1-866-860-0900. There are people who will be delighted to answer your questions. Also, you can find out more about our international seminar schedule on our website at www.brandonbays.com.

May your chosen journey be filled with the joy of self-discovery and wholeness, and may you uncover the extraordinary beauty of your own soul.

Acknowledgments

I could not possibly name all the people who have contributed to *The Journey*, but I would like to express my gratitude individually to some of the people who played a *specific* role in my journey to health—my close friends who tirelessly believed in me and supported me through it—Debra Angeletti, Skip Lackey, Catherine Curry, "Kabir" Jeremy Geffen, and Mark and Elaine Thomas. My heartfelt thanks to Don, my former husband, who constantly urged me onward in my spiritual unfolding; to my daughter Kelley, for her wisdom and trust; and my dear friends Tony and Becky Robbins, who held out the certain belief that I would heal. My special thanks to David Marshall for his generous and constant support, both as a friend and for his expert advice in developing The Journey seminars, and to Neidda his wife for her loving care throughout the writing of this book.

I'm especially grateful to Vicki St. George, for not only being there for me as a dear friend, but also for generously helping with the preliminary edit of this book. And to Carole Tonkinson, whose own love of Truth made her the perfect editor to work with in creating the original edition of this book. A special thanks to Nada, Catherine and Peter Whitfield, and Marlisse Karlin for kindly helping me get the first Journey Seminars off the ground.

My gratitude to my mother for her belief in me, and for imparting to me her great love of beauty and nature.

With all my heart, I would like to thank the teachers and therapists who have inspired me, especially Surja Jessup. However, this book would become an encyclopedia of names if I were to list all those who have had a profound impact on both my life and this work. In the fields of NLP, NAC, iridology, acupressure, herbology, nutrition, kinesiology, medical hypnosis, psycho-neuro immunology, psychology and personal growth, every teacher has given me some gem. There is one man, however, I feel must be mentioned—Dr. Deepak Chopra. Through his extensive research, he has inspired millions with the certain knowledge that cellular healing is possible. And also a thank you to Candace Pert for her groundbreaking research on cellular healing.

More people than I could possibly name have supported The Journey in getting the message out. A special thanks to Lipi and Darren Bagshaw, Ross Marlow and Shirley Roche, Teresa Curren, Jonathan Austin, Nick Williams, Carol Marples-Kemble, Suzy Greaves, and Mark and Elizabeth Riminton for their dedication to helping others on their paths of growth. A special thanks to Melanie Boyd and Tim Forbess, President of the National Foundation of Alternative Medicine, for their extraordinary efforts on behalf of The Journey.

More recently, my heartfelt gratitude to Anne Edelstein for her integrity, enthusiasm, and exquisite sensitivity in championing the book. And my love and gratitude to "The Journey Team," Gaby, Cliff, Trish, Debs, Laurie, Amba, Jess, Suzi, Sarah, and Paul for their constant love and support.

My heart is deeply grateful to those awakened teachers who woke me up to the Truth of who I am, and who have given their lives in service to Truth—pointing to the greatness within us all—Krishnamurti, Gangaji, Catherine Ingram, and Ramana Maharishi. My deepest heartfelt gratitude to Gurumayi for the initial awakening, and I will forever be indebted to HWL Poonja for "smashing the pot," destroying the concept of separate identity, giving the direct realization of Self—the essence of this book. May my life be lived as a never-ending prayer of gratitude in service to this that is revealed in their presence.

And my most profound thanks to my partner, Kevin, whose own devotion to Truth saw me through the creation and editing of this book. He passionately believed in the book's message, and his desire to serve humankind made him hold the book up to the magnifying light of Truth. He made certain it had the highest standards of purity and honesty.

Thank you to the thousands who have used The Journey to transform their lives, and to the courageous and generous souls whose inspiring stories fill this book (some of their names have been changed to protect their privacy).

Most important, my gratitude to Truth itself for awakening me to the love and greatness within.